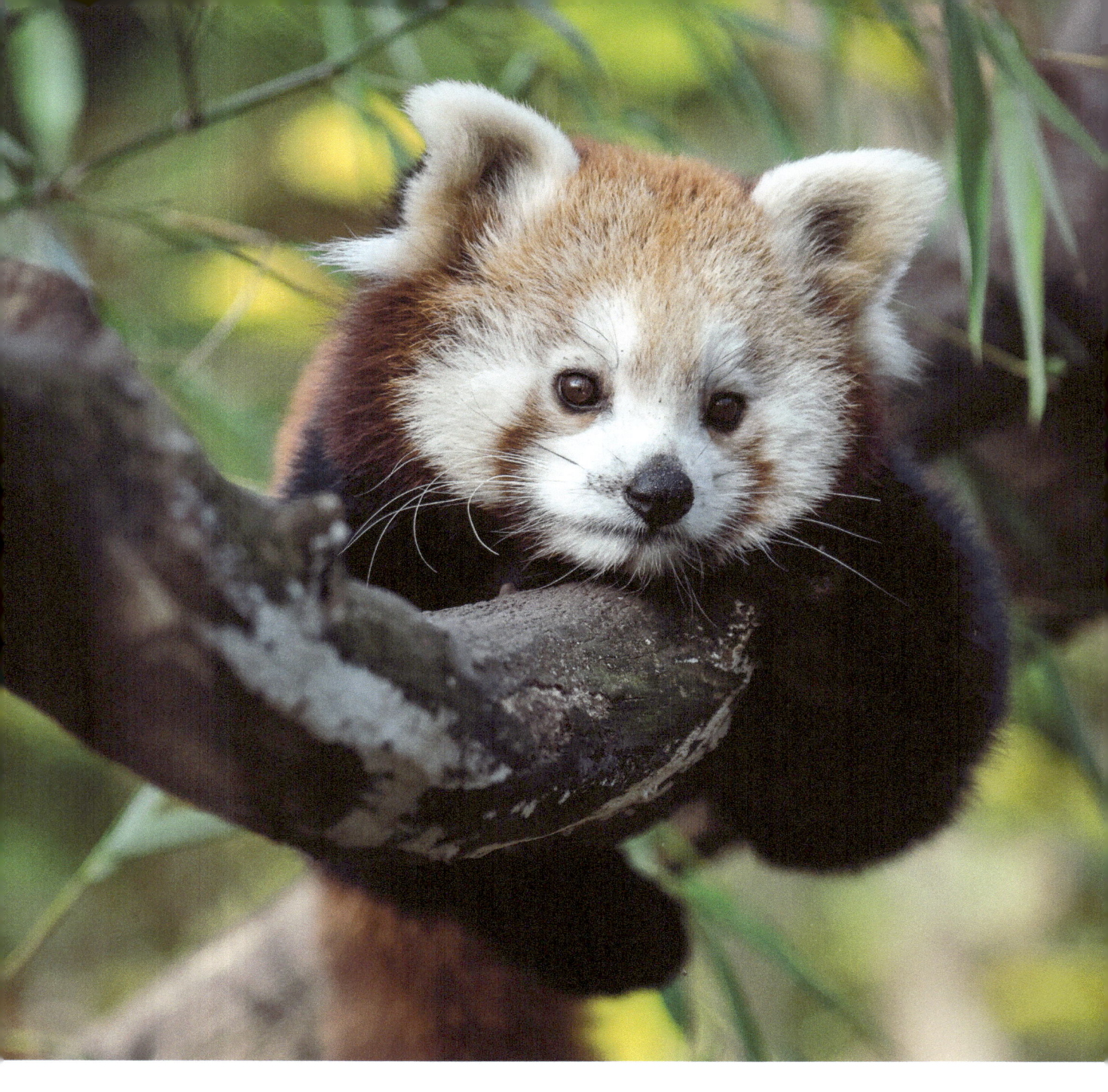

A red panda

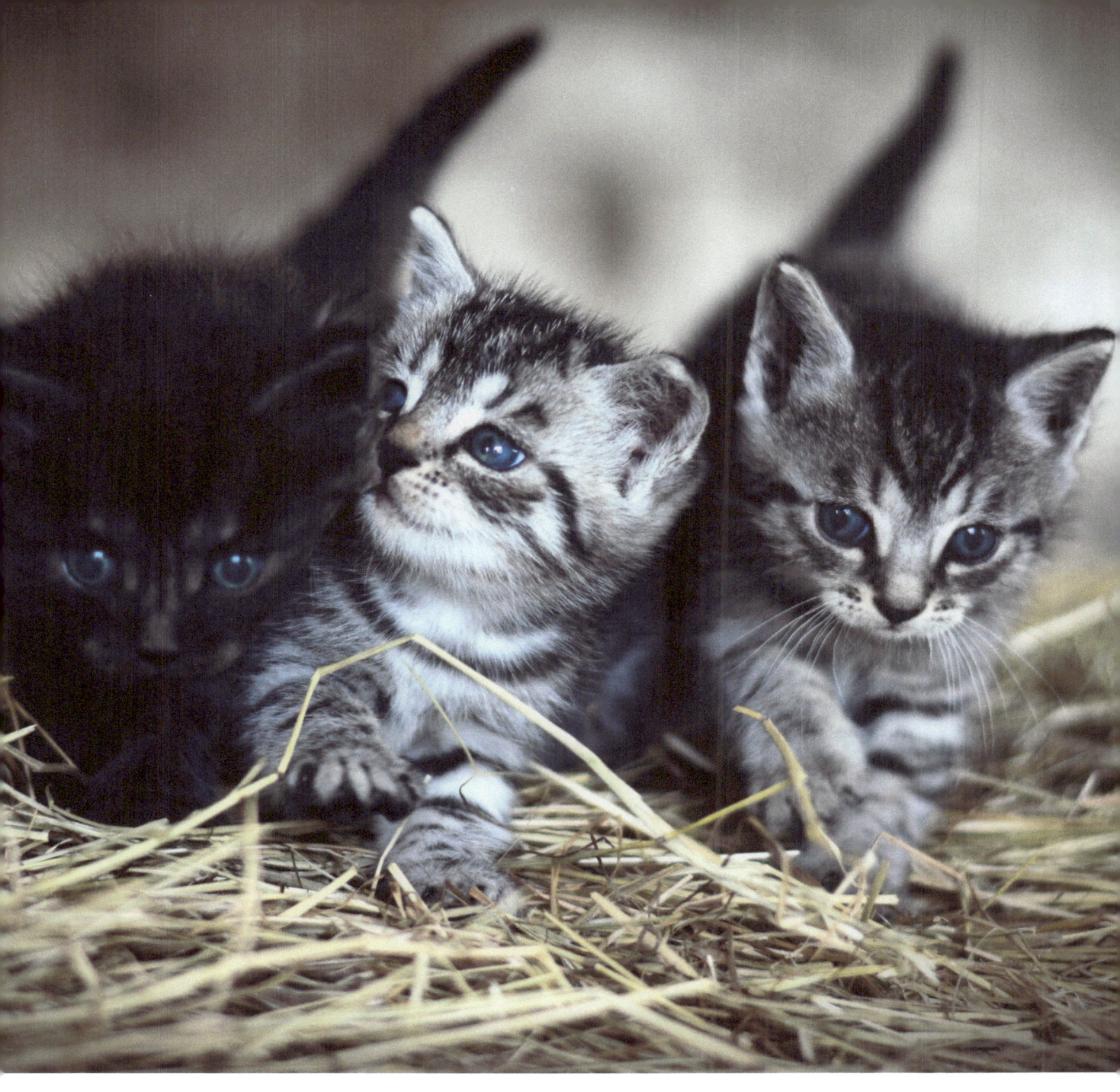

Three kittens

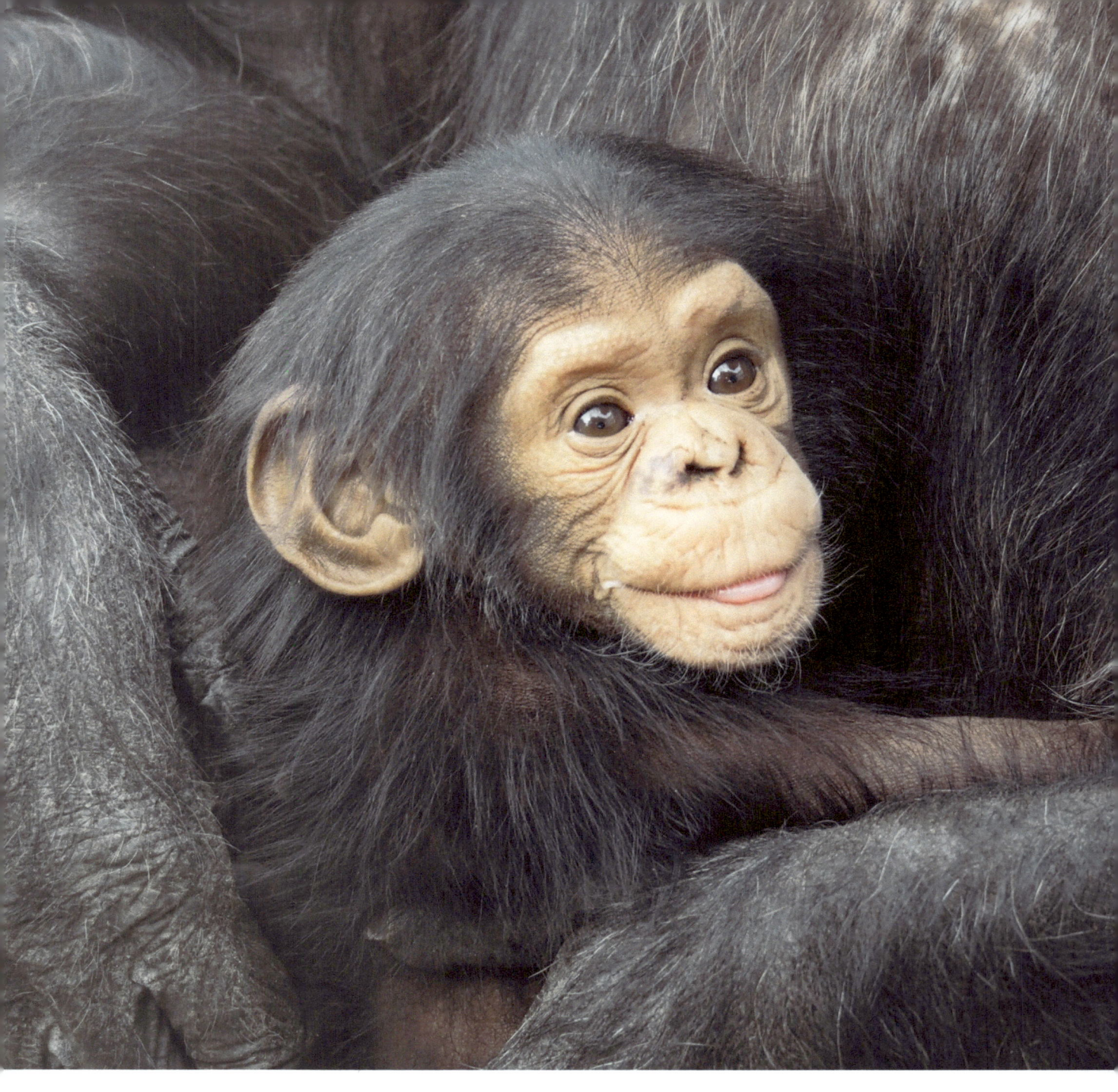

A chimpanzee

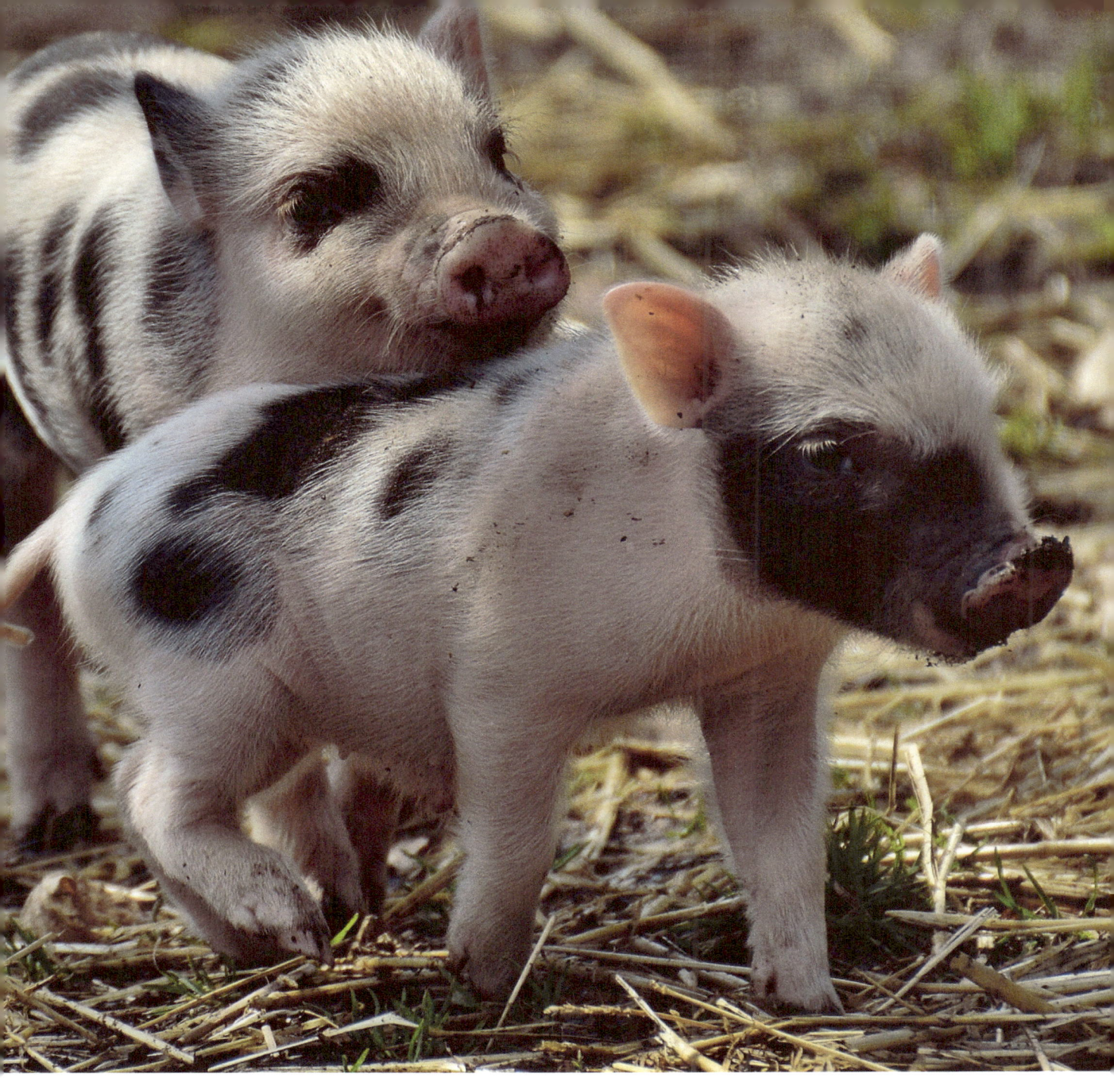

Two piglets

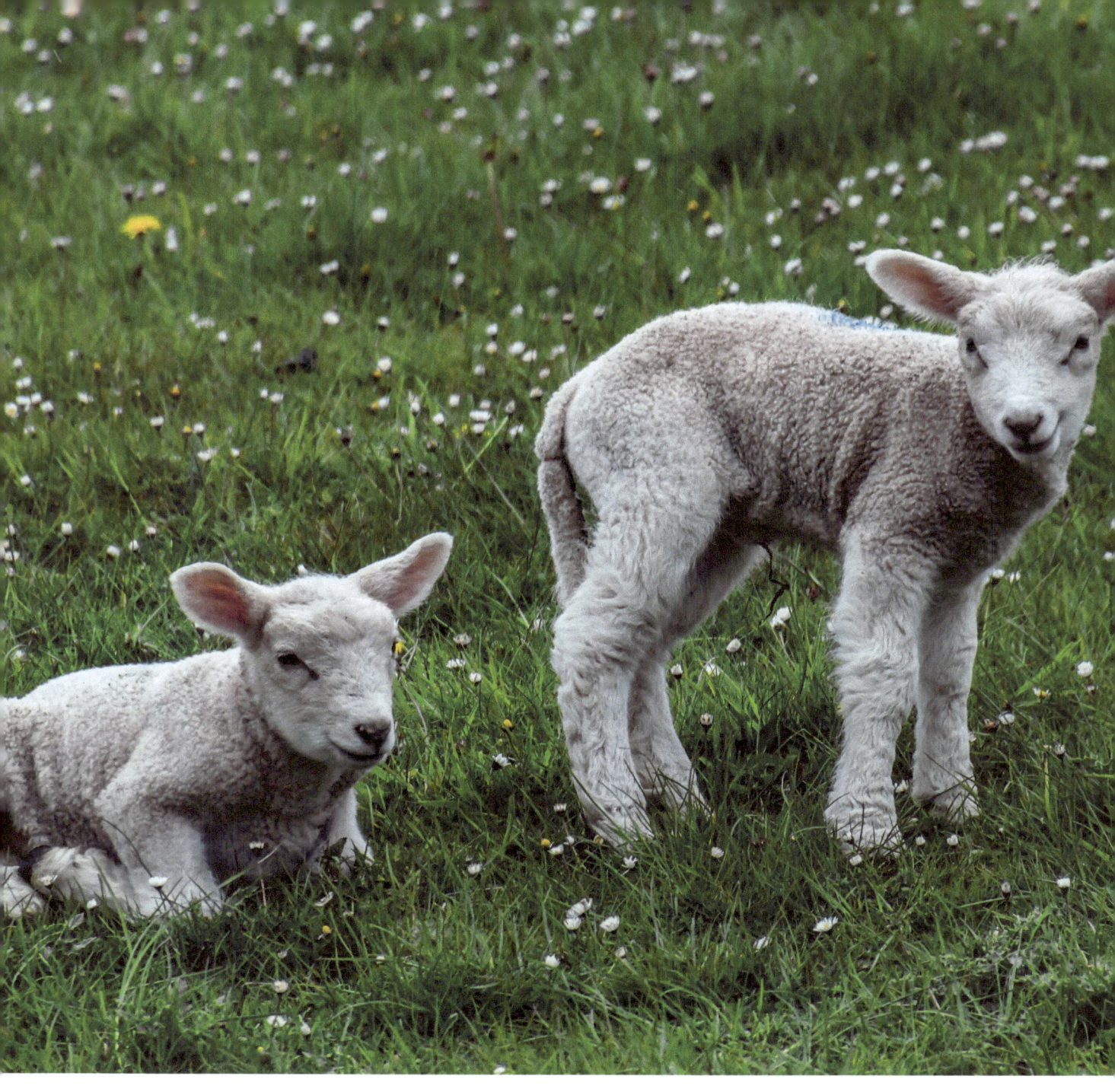

Two lambs

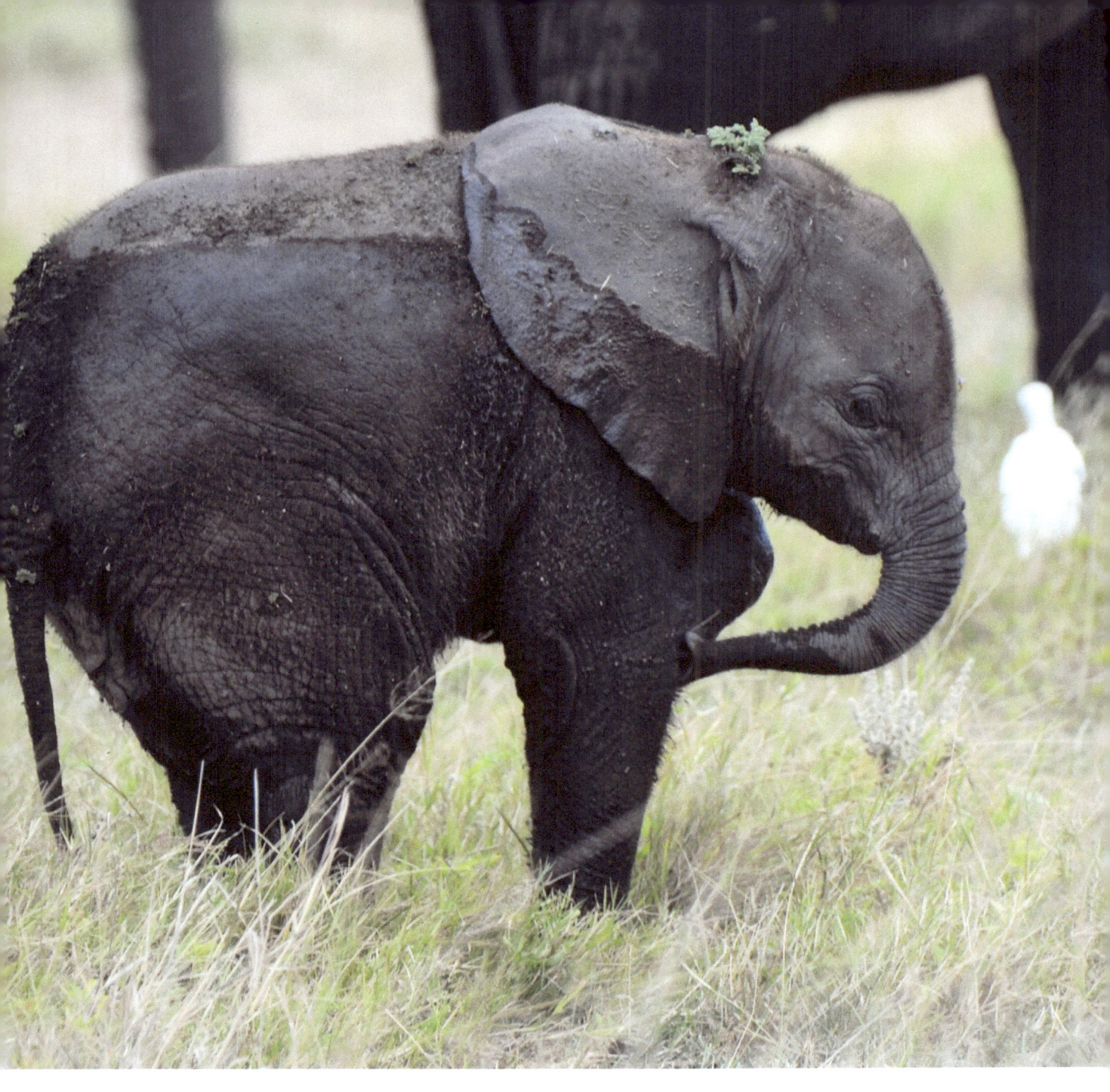

An elephant

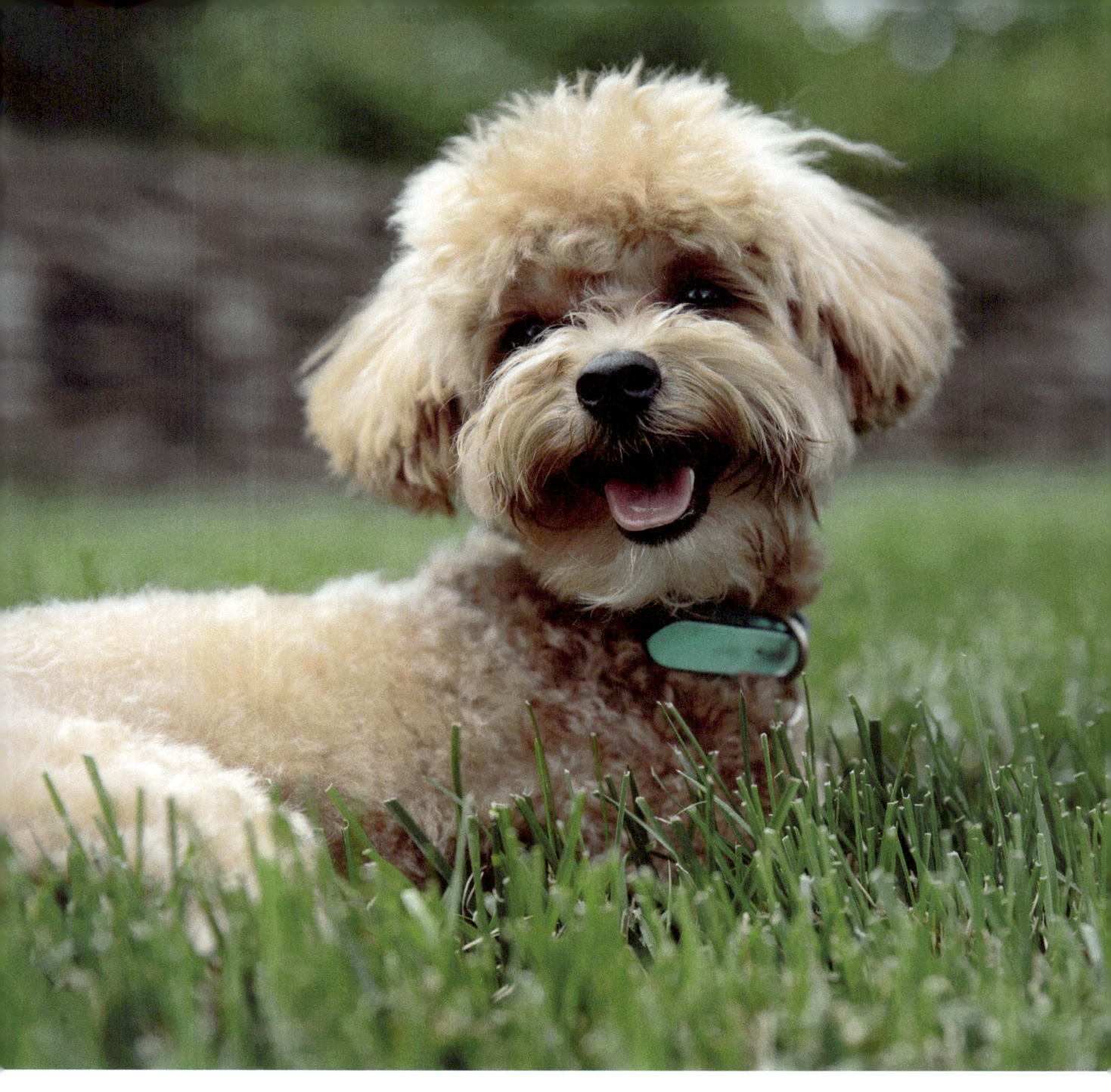

A puppy

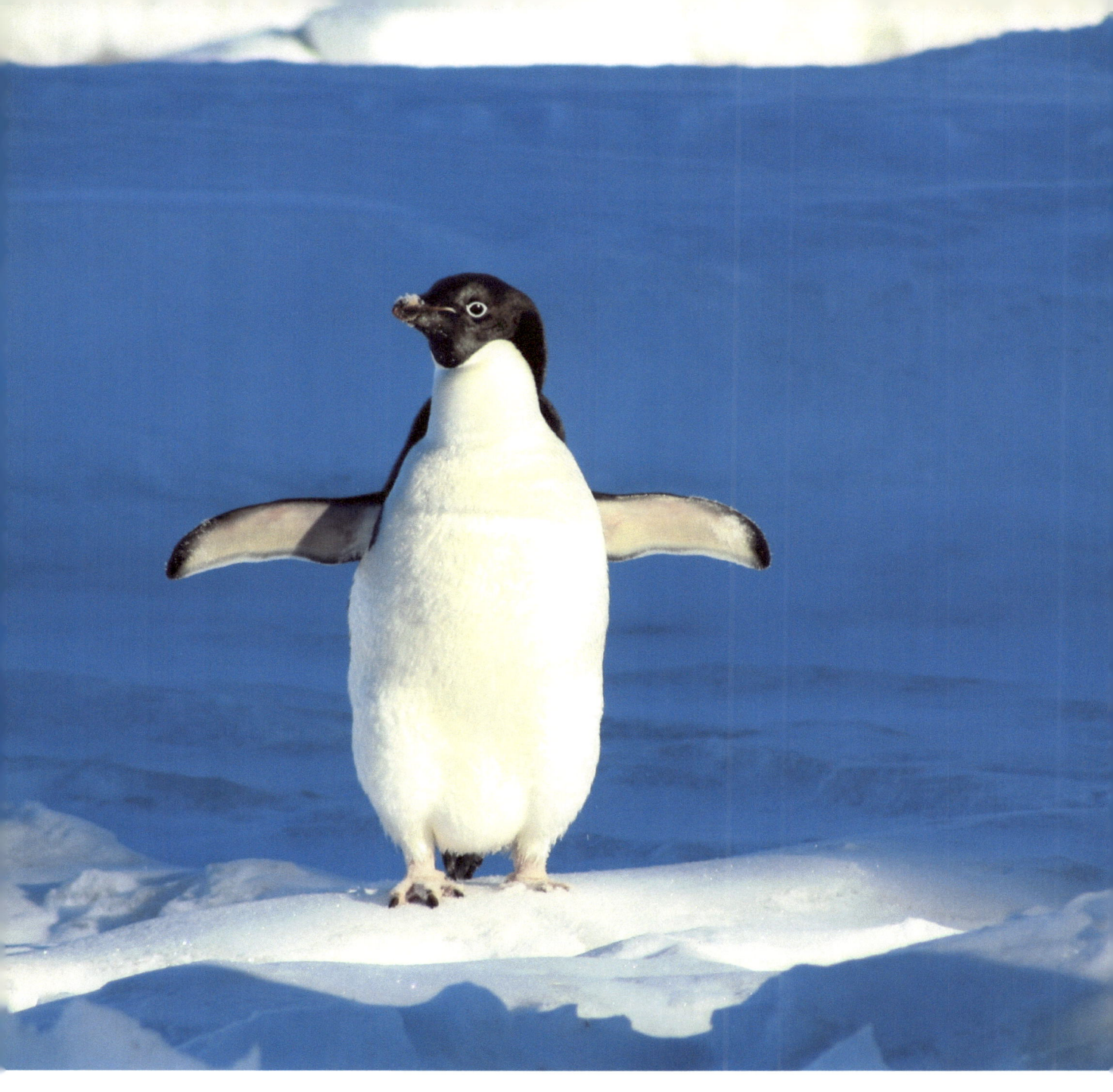

A penguin

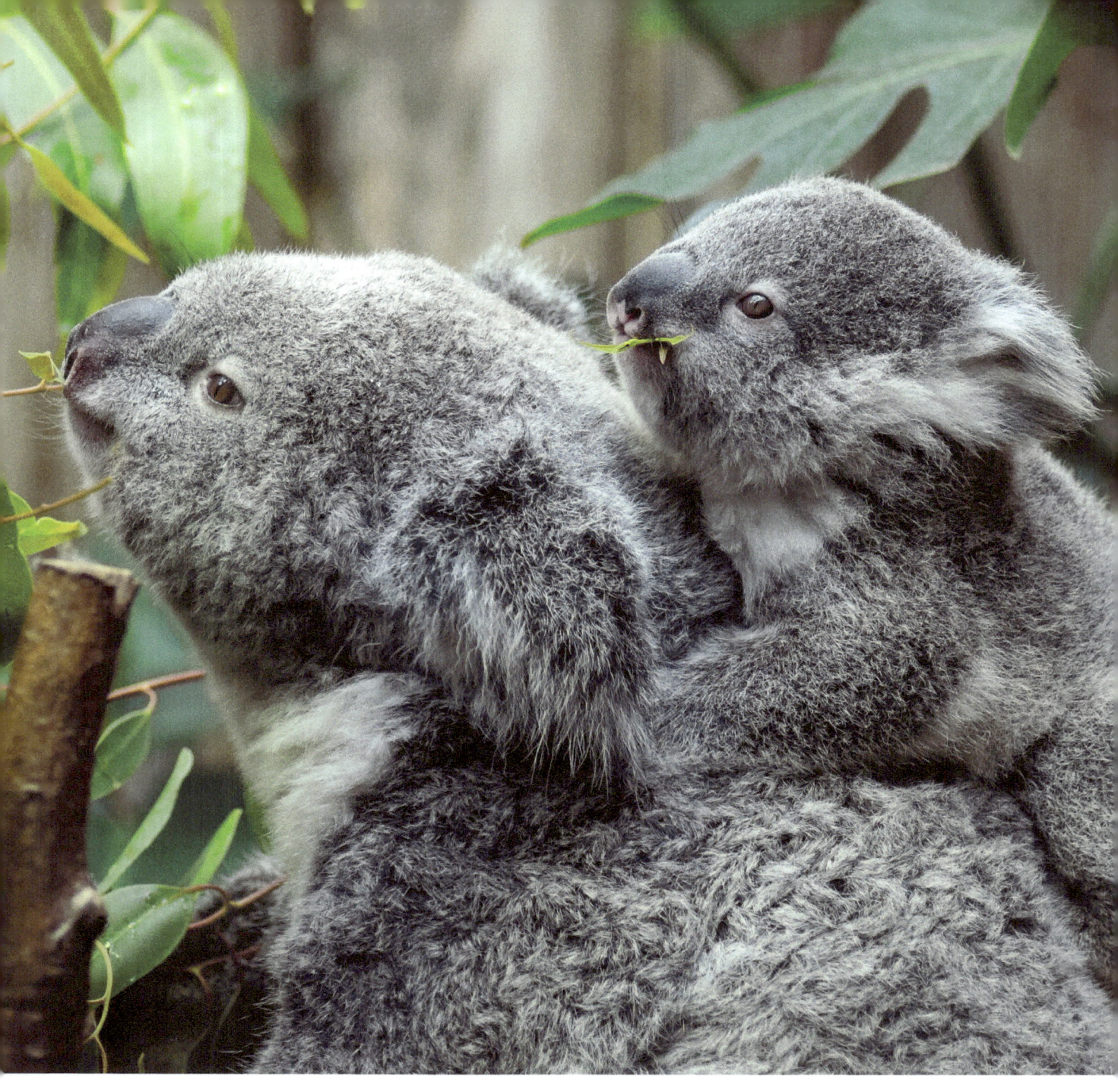

Two koalas

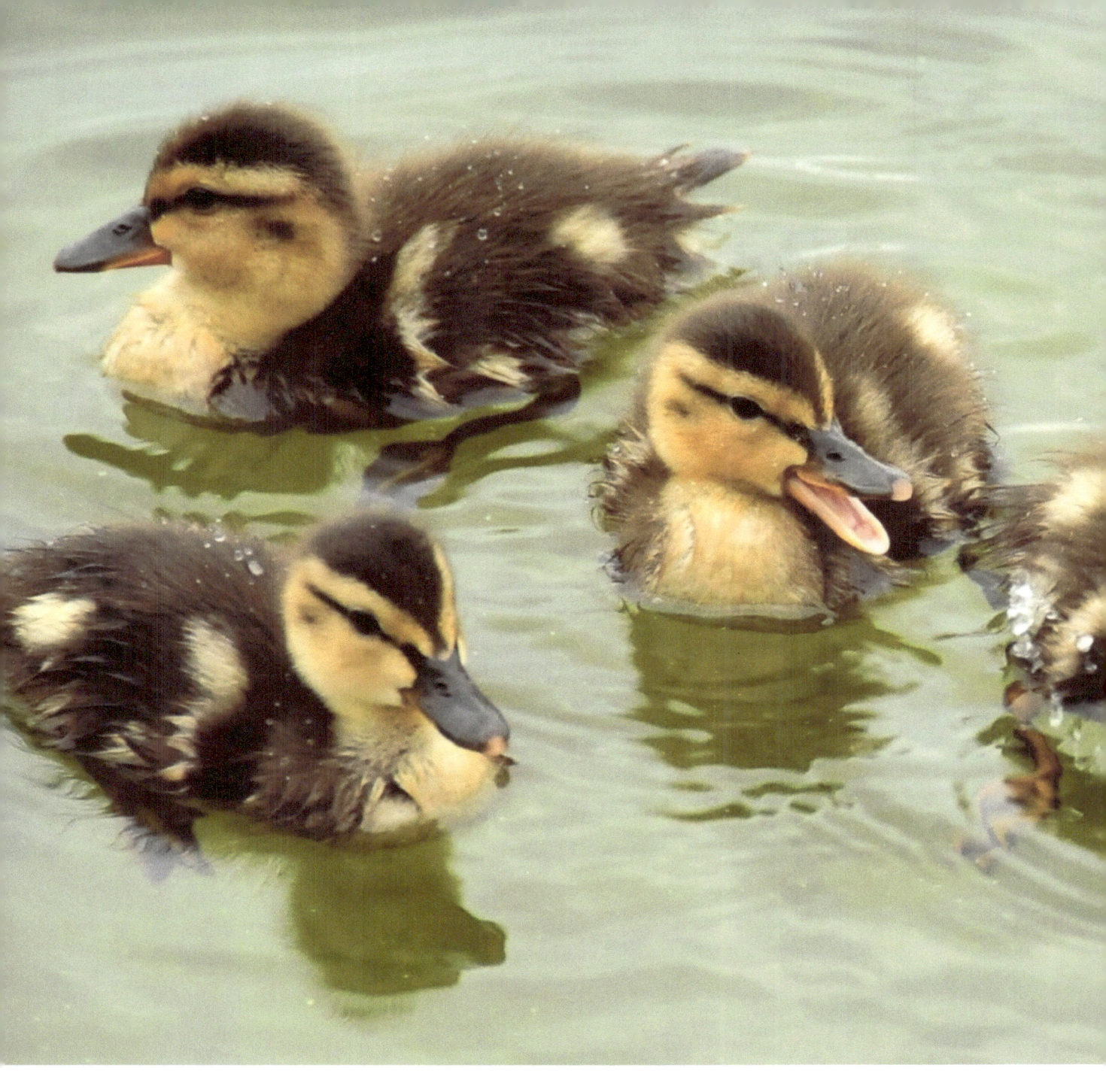

Ducklings

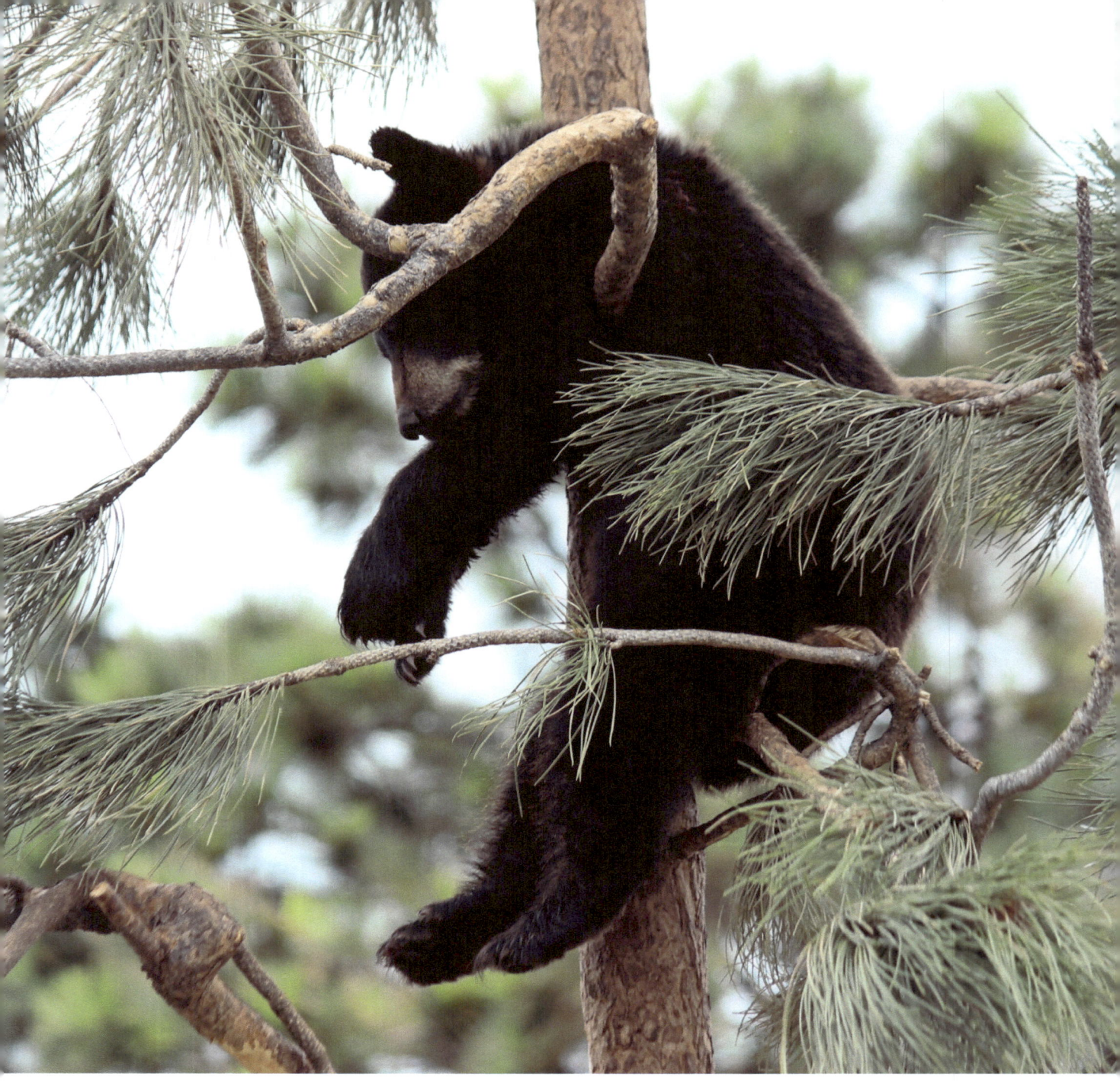

A bear

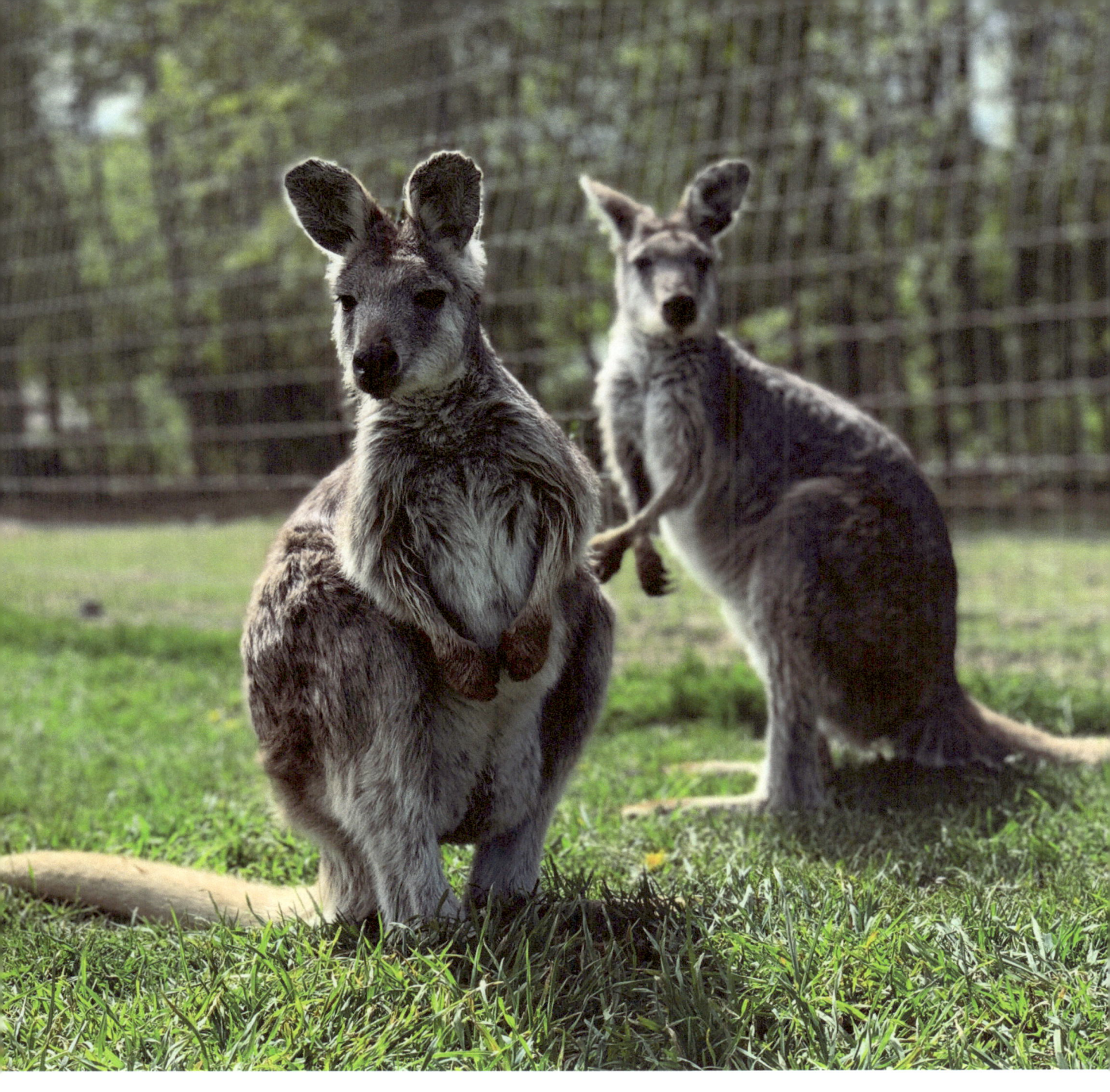

Two wallabies

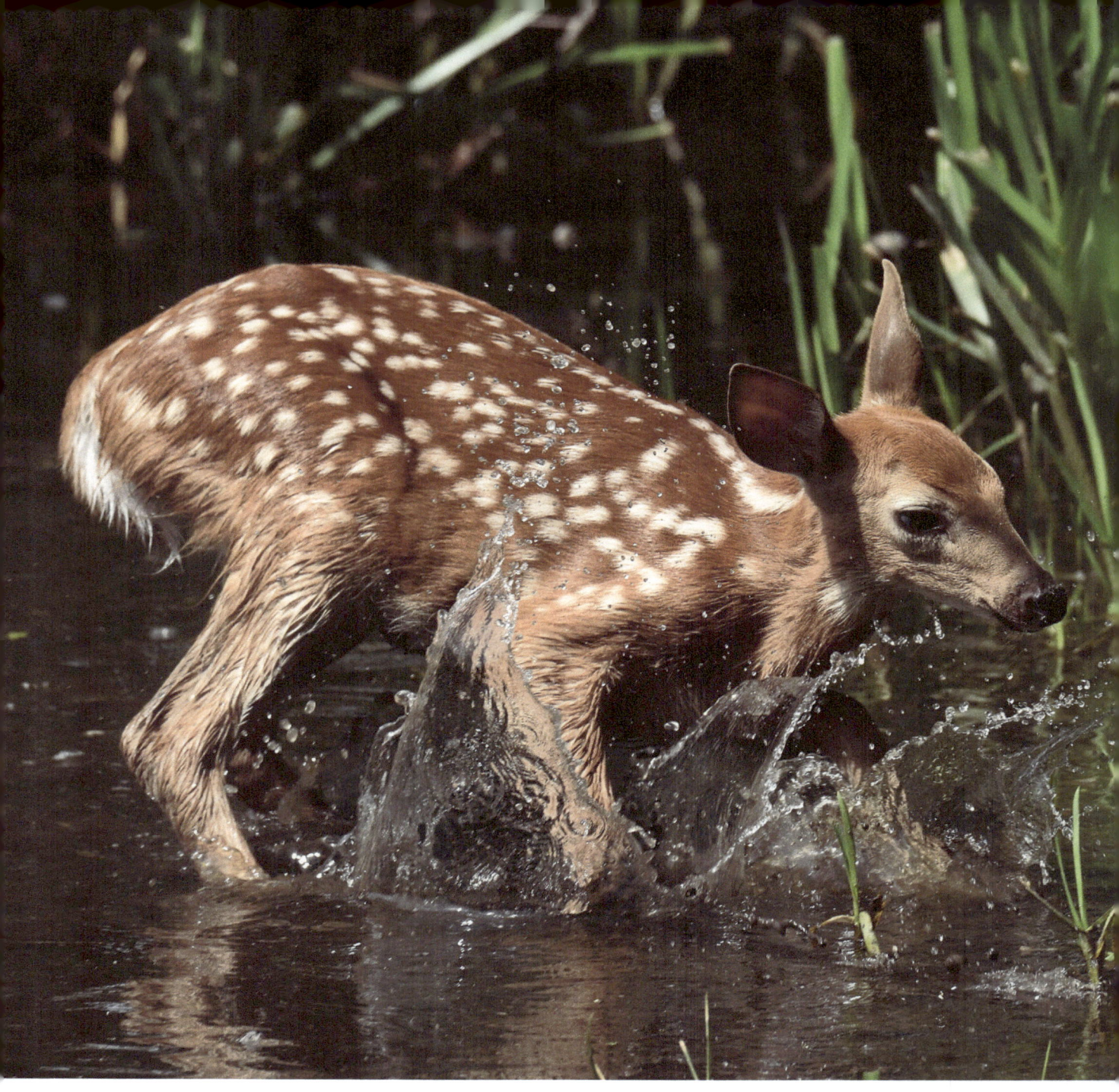

A fawn

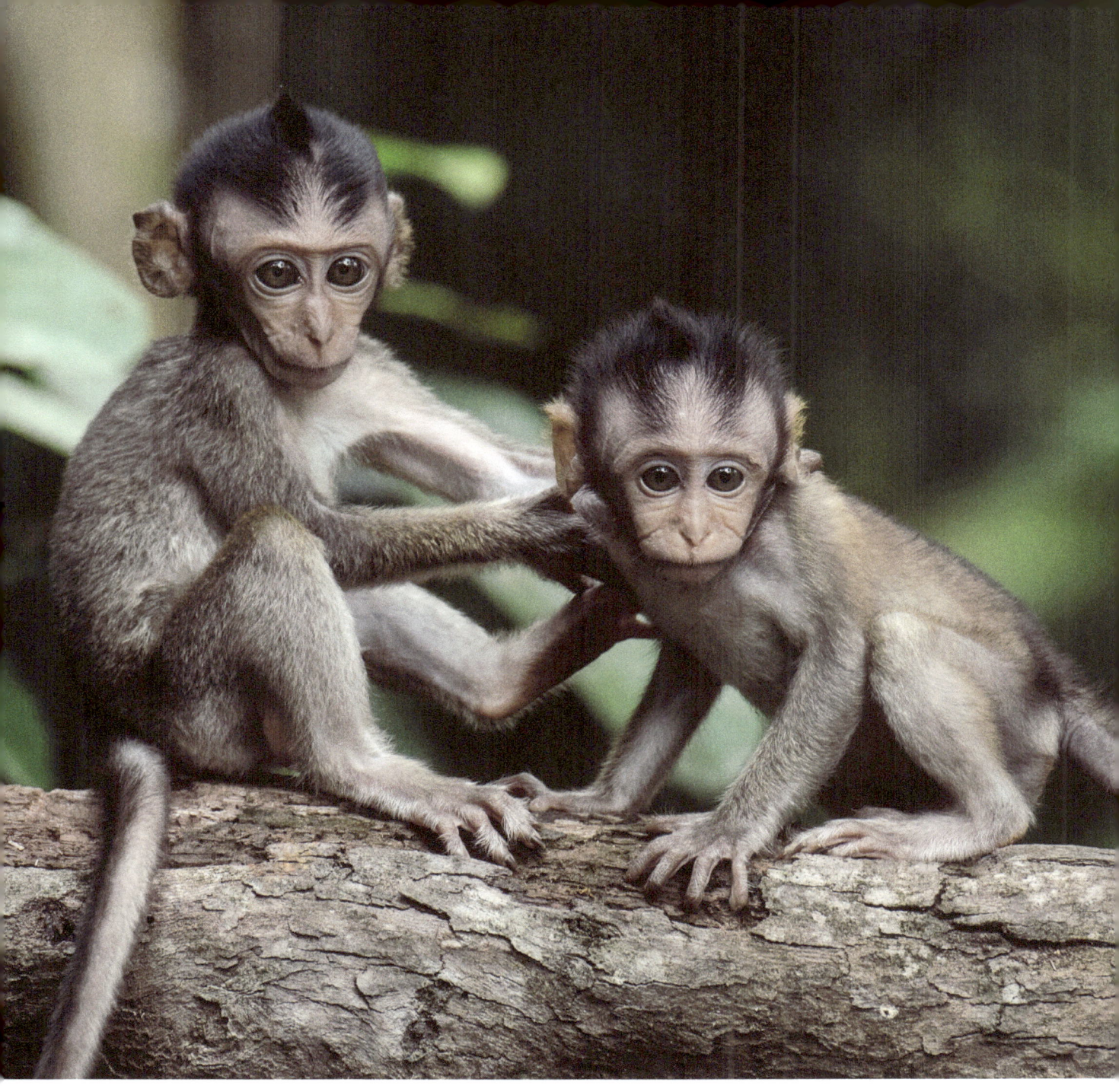

Two monkeys

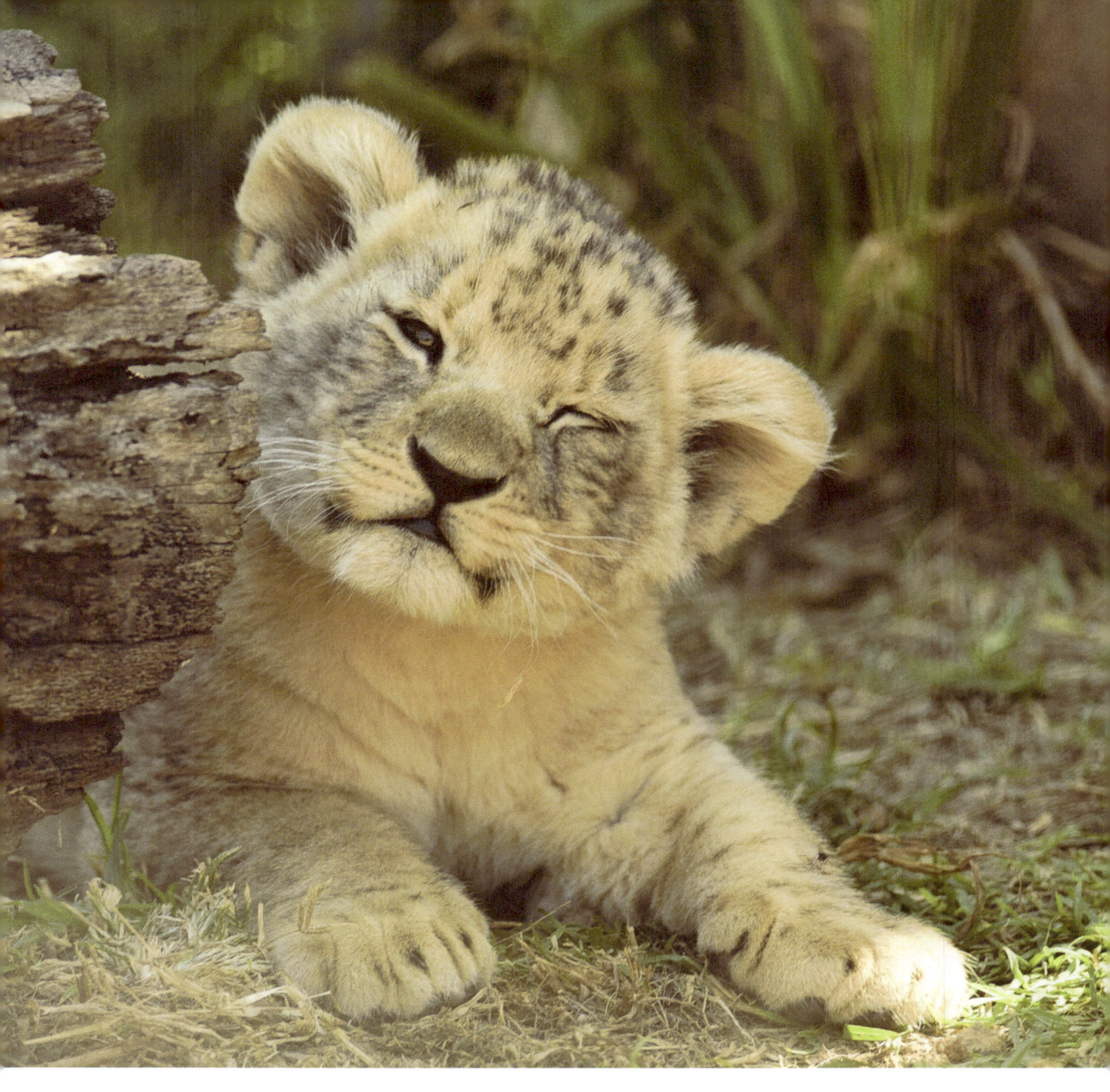

A lion cub

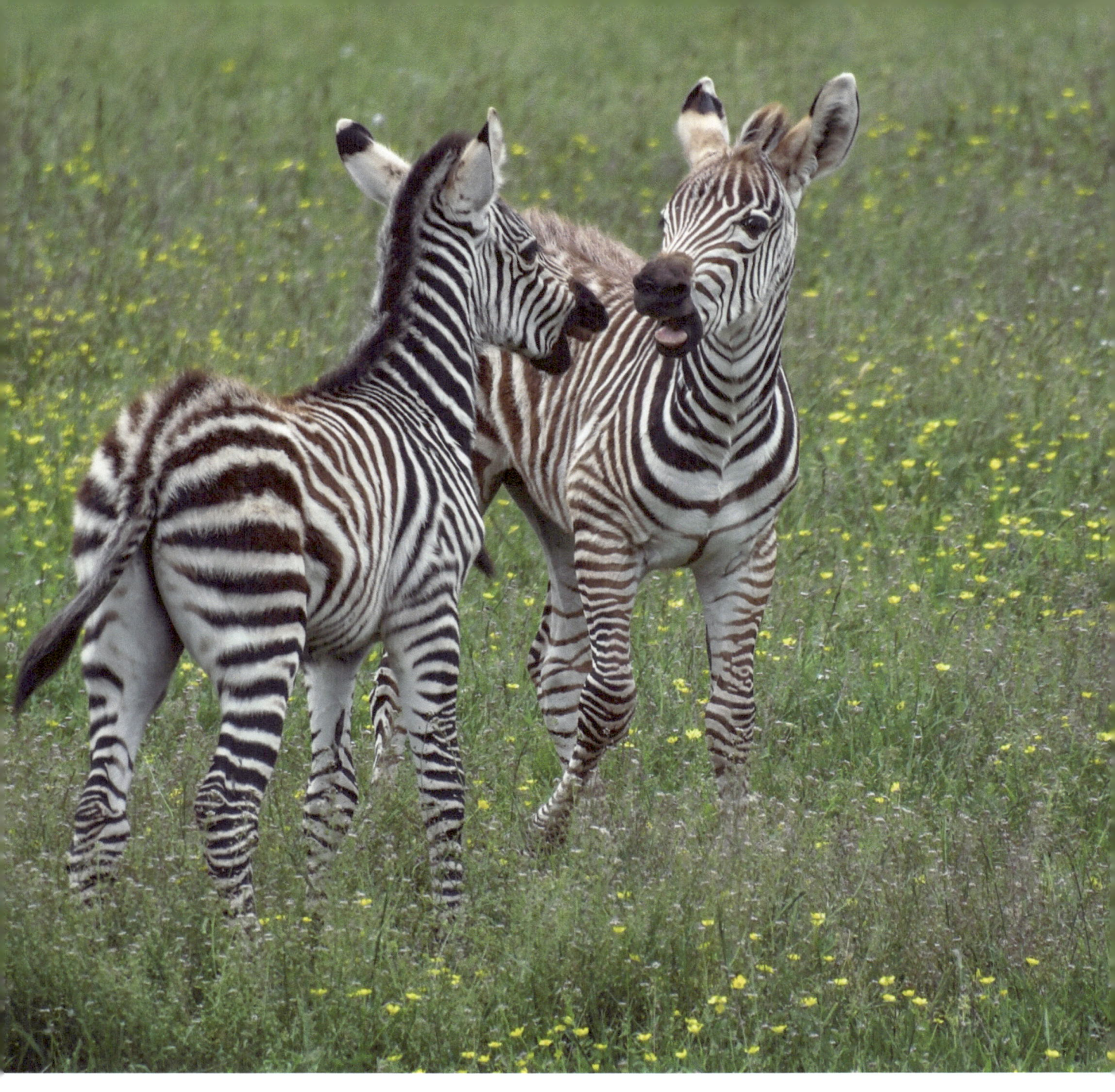

Two zebras

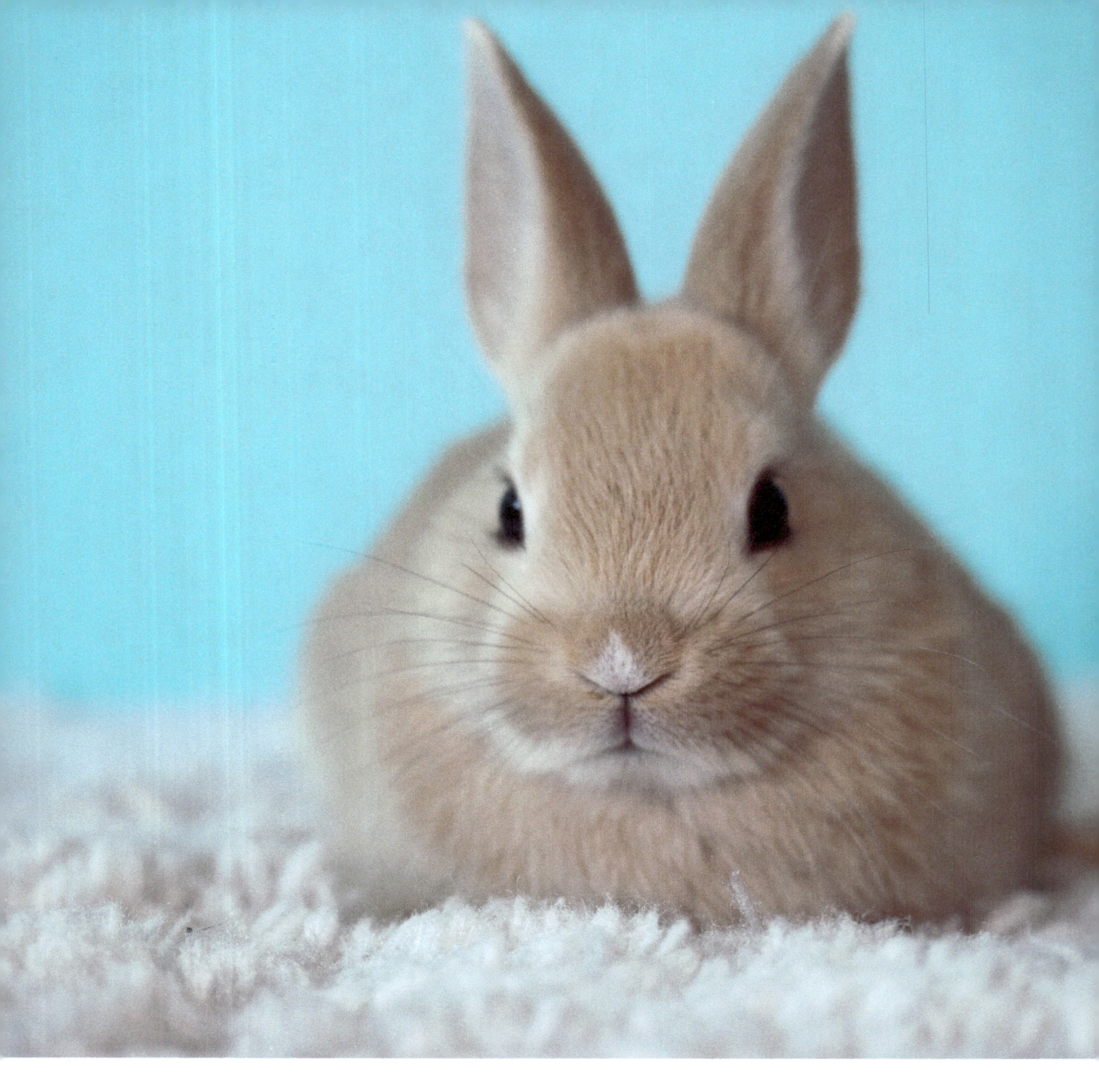

A bunny

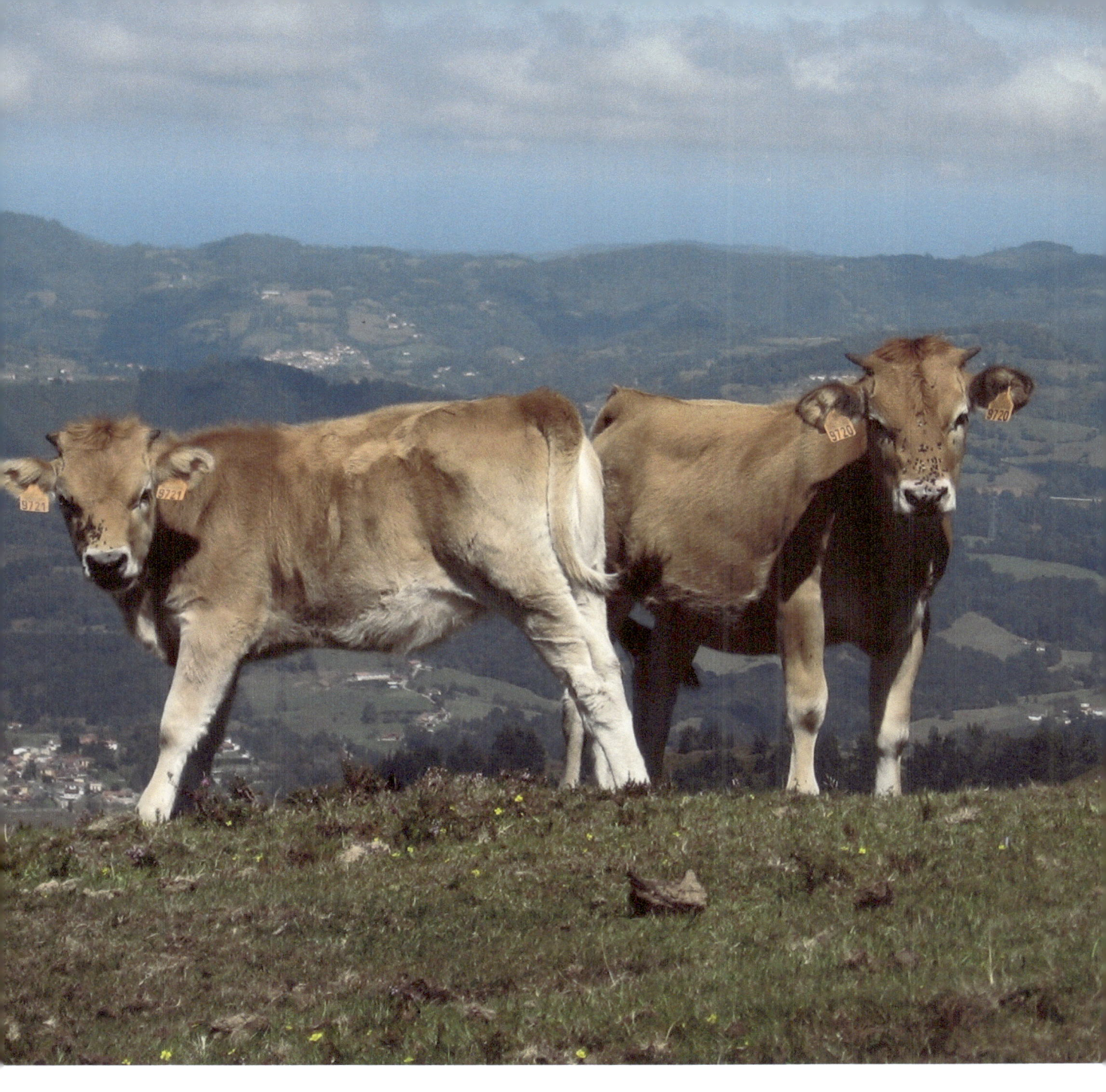

Two calves

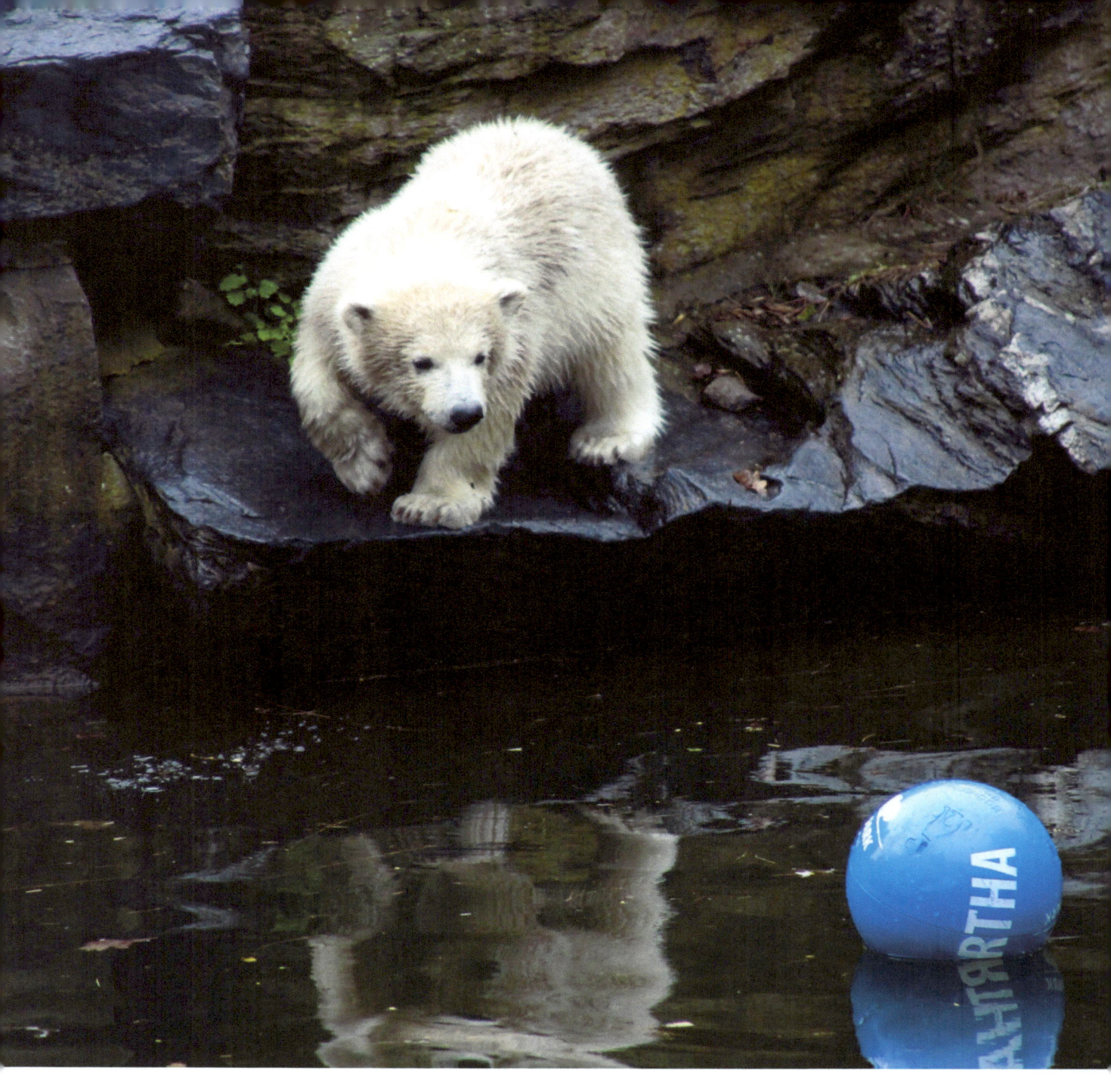

A polar bear

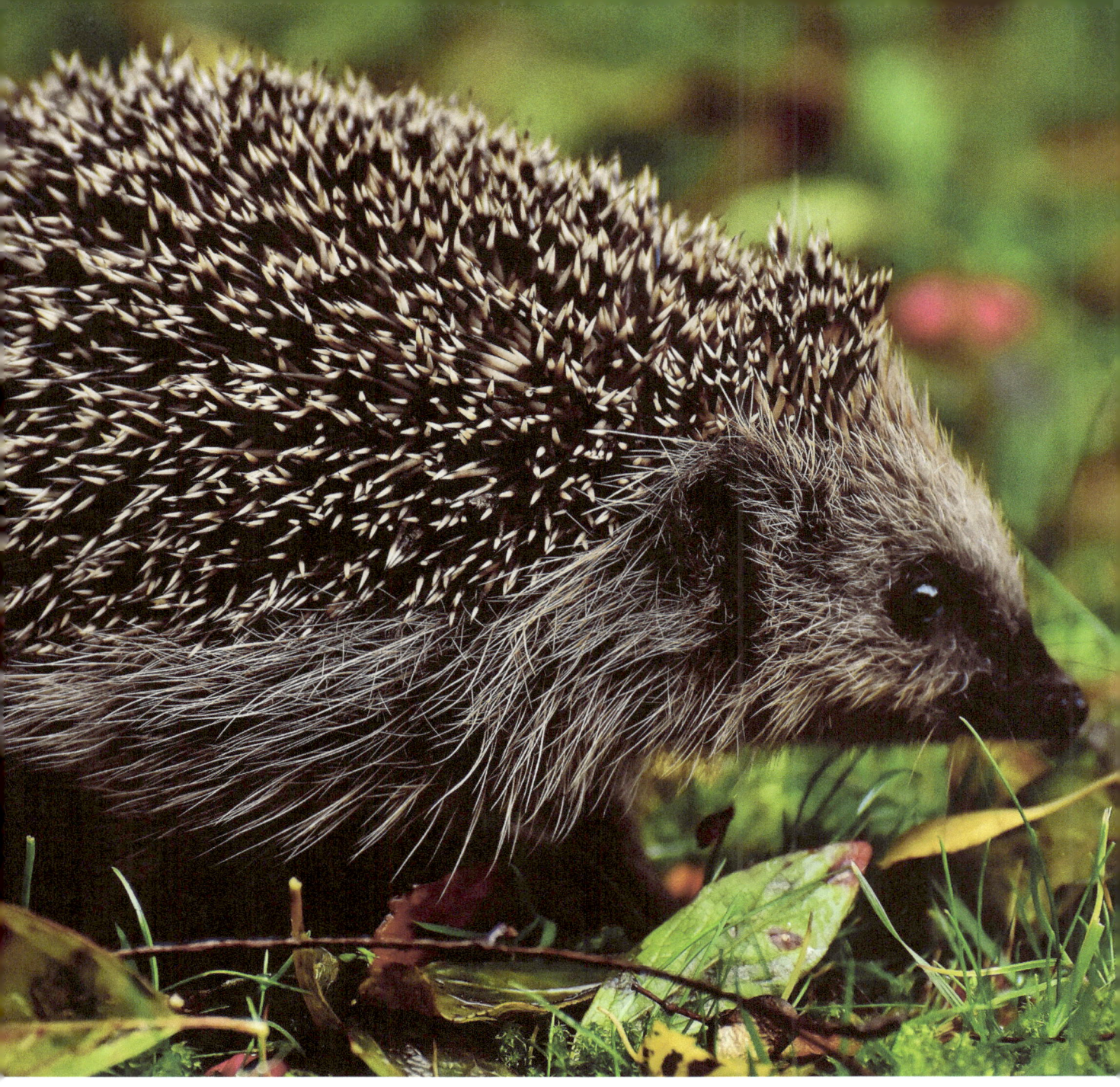

A hedgehog

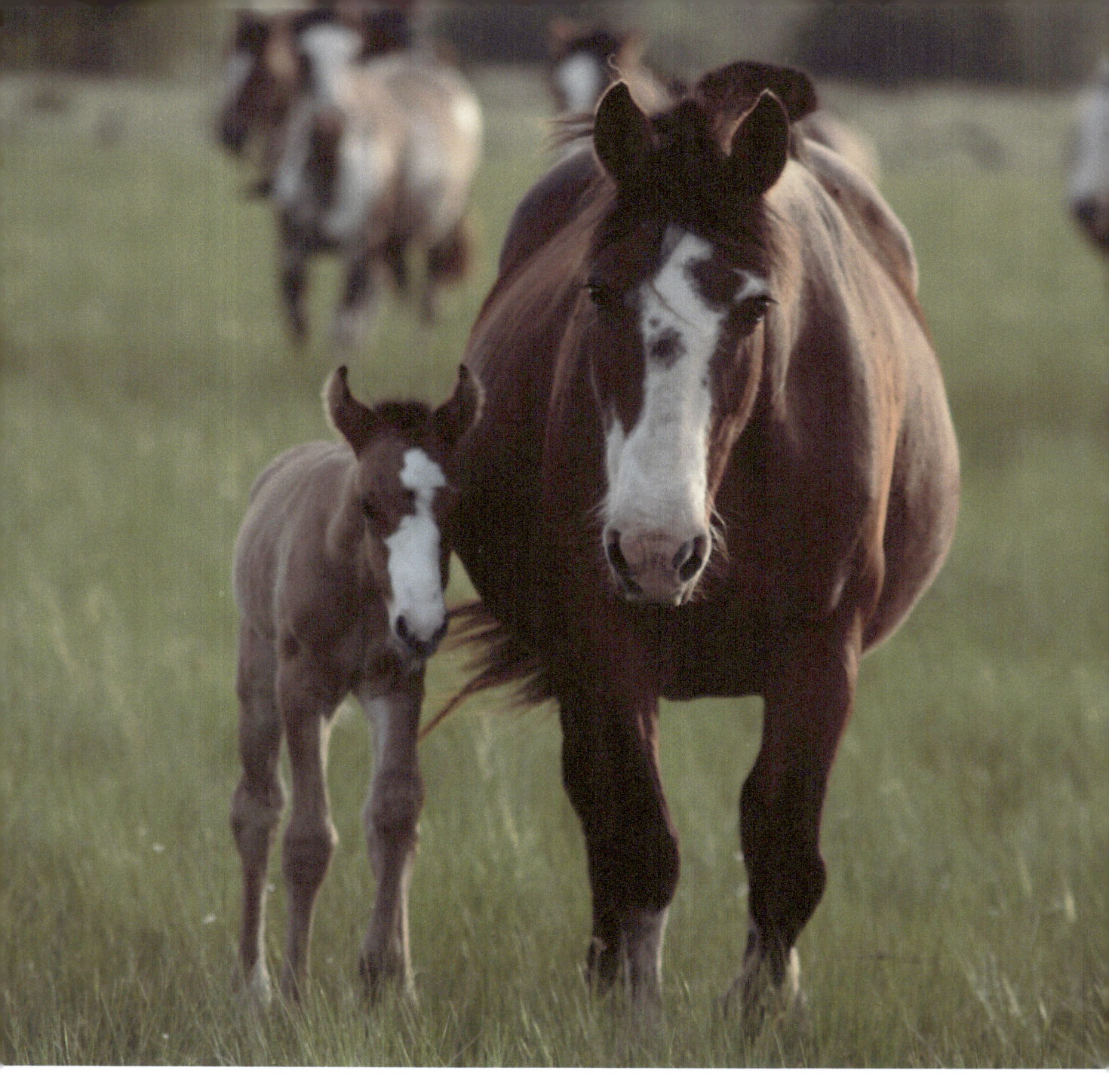

Two horses

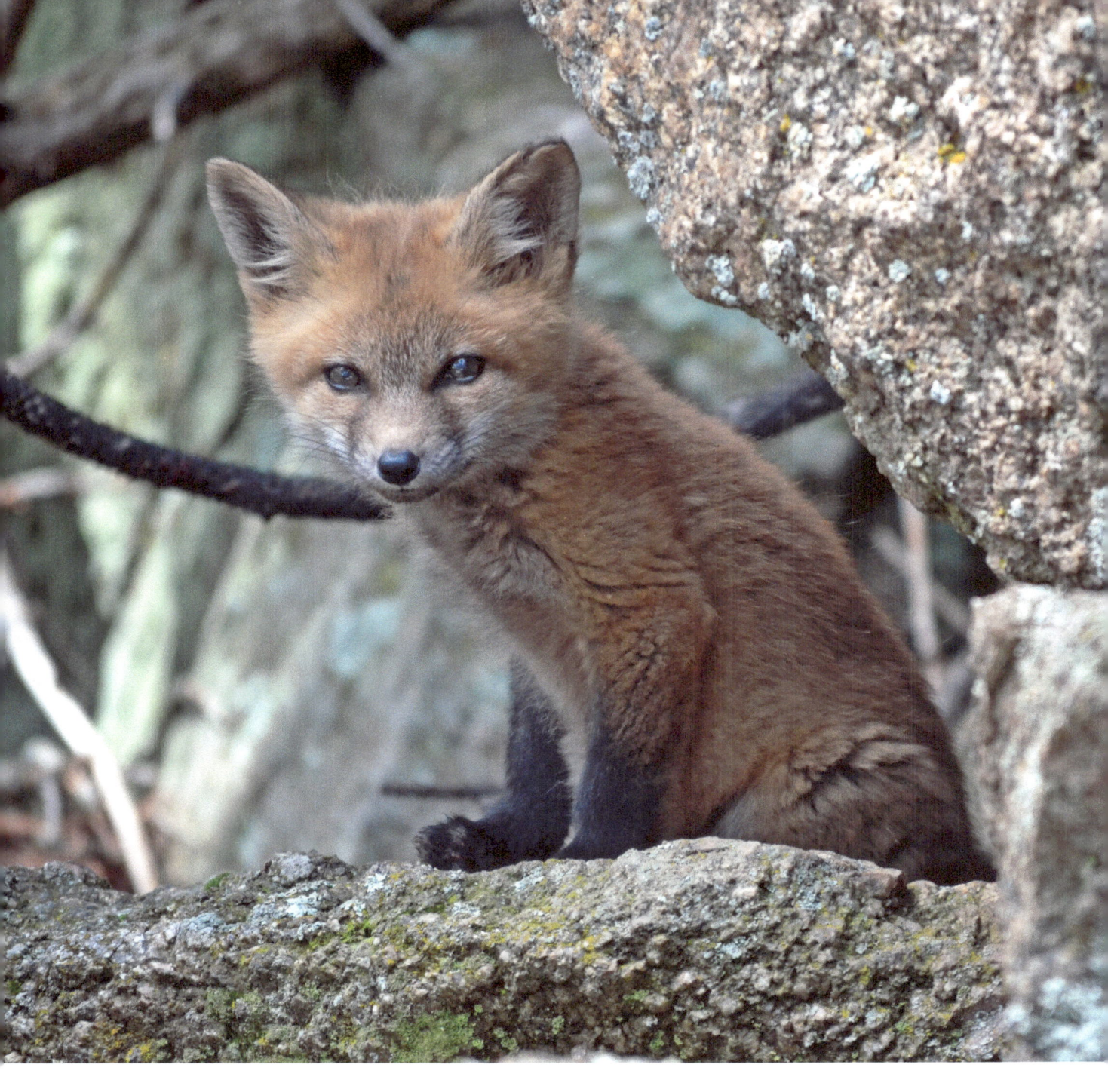

A fox

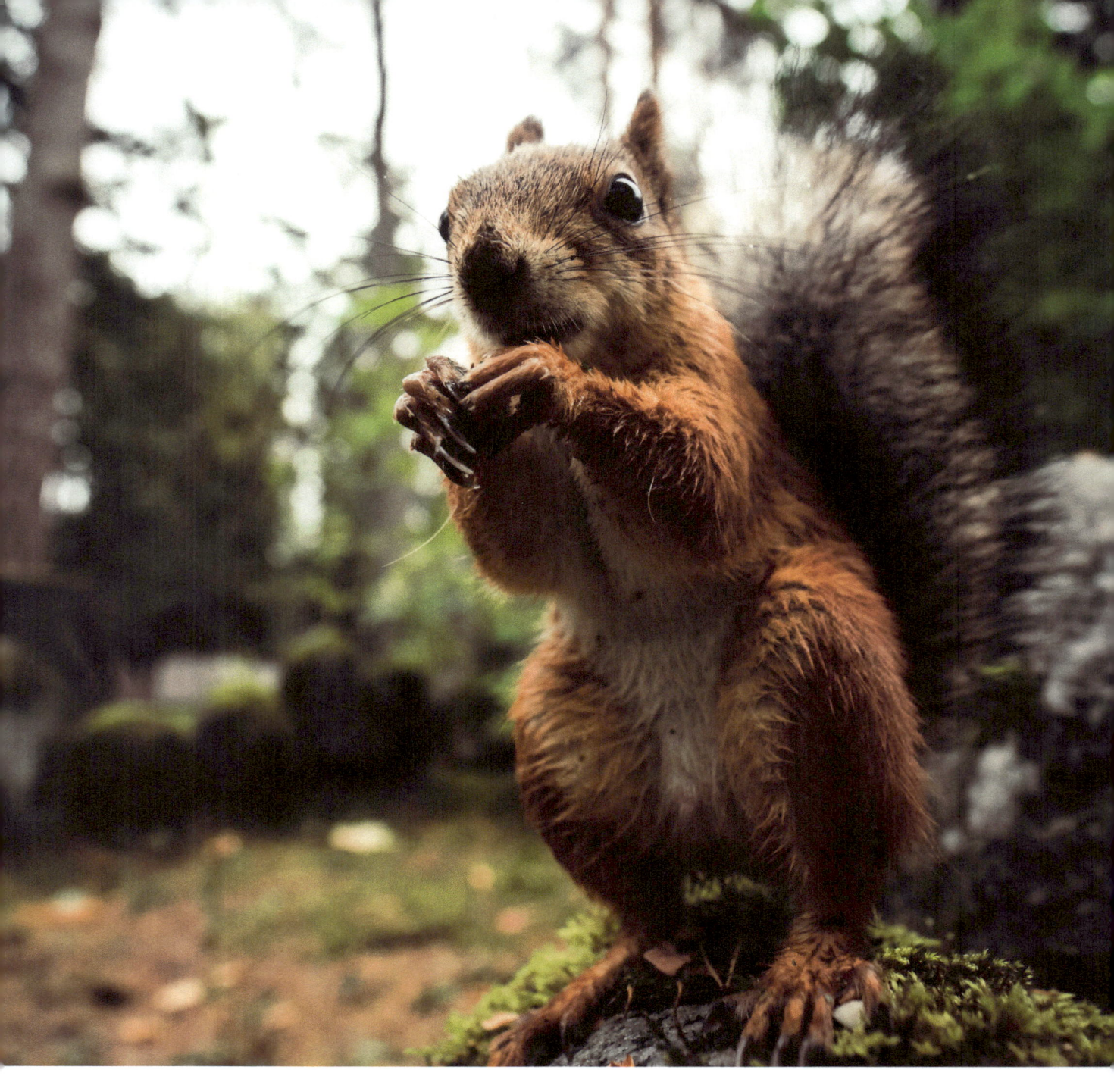

A squirrel

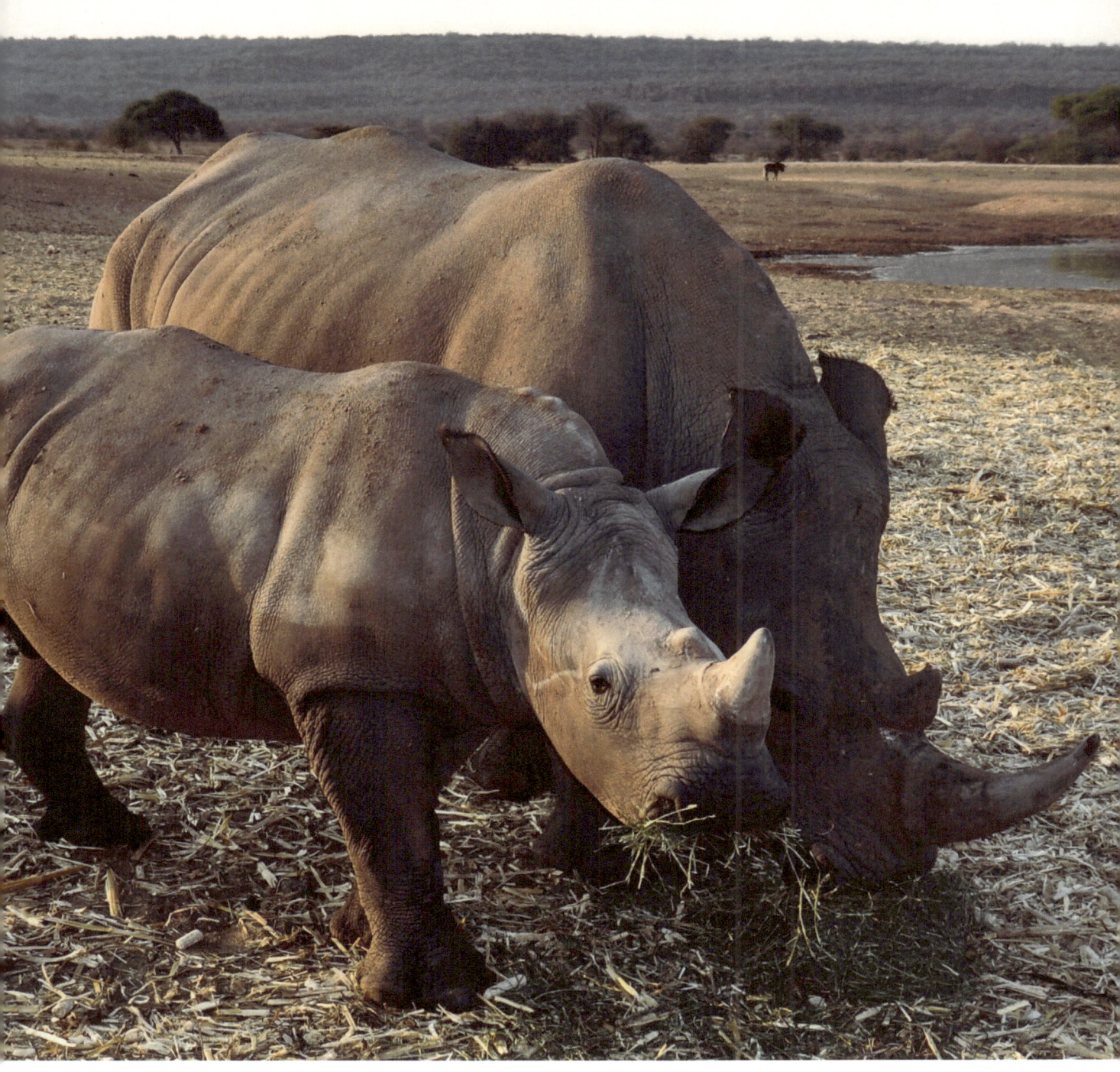

Two rhinos

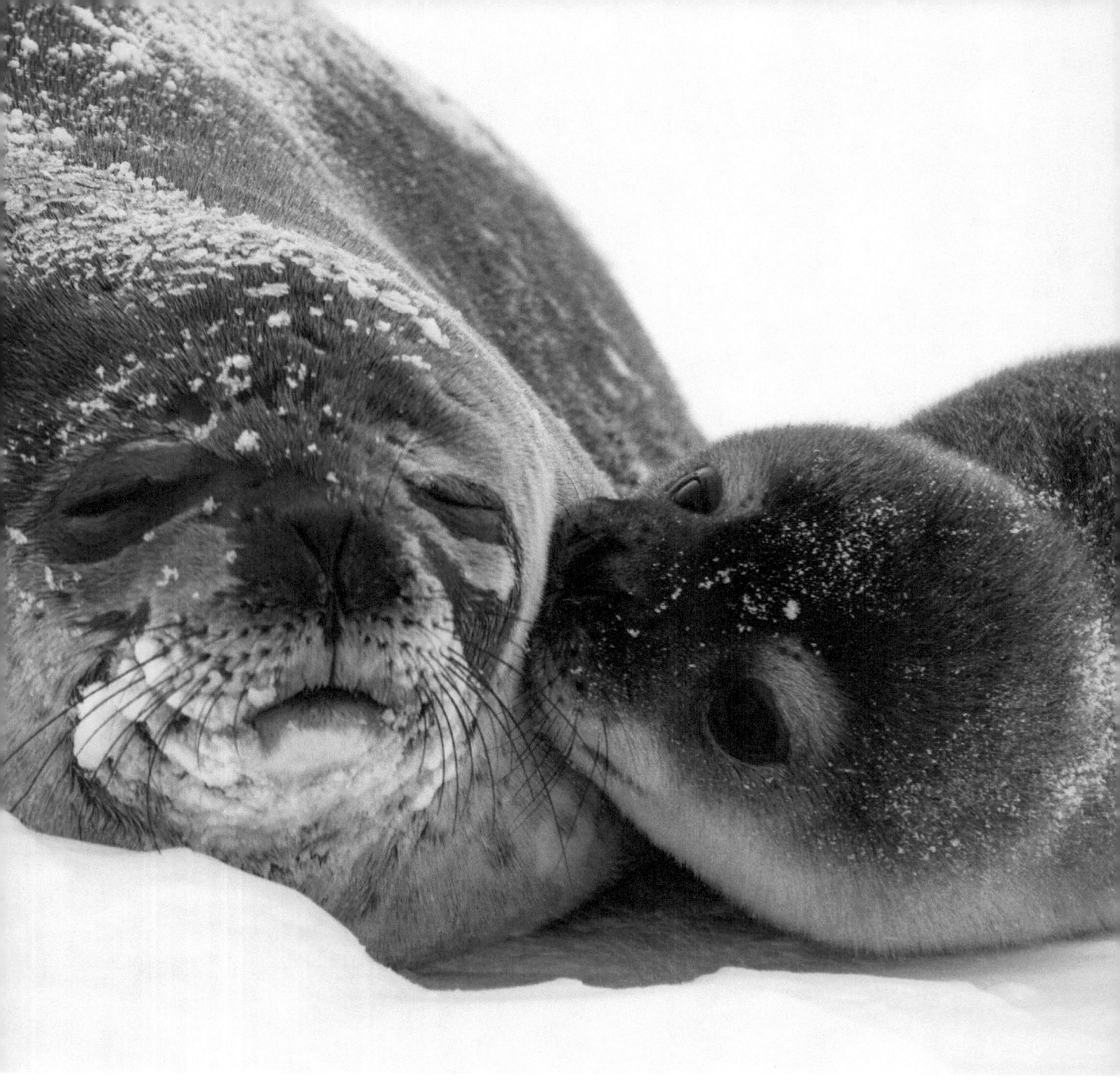

Two seals

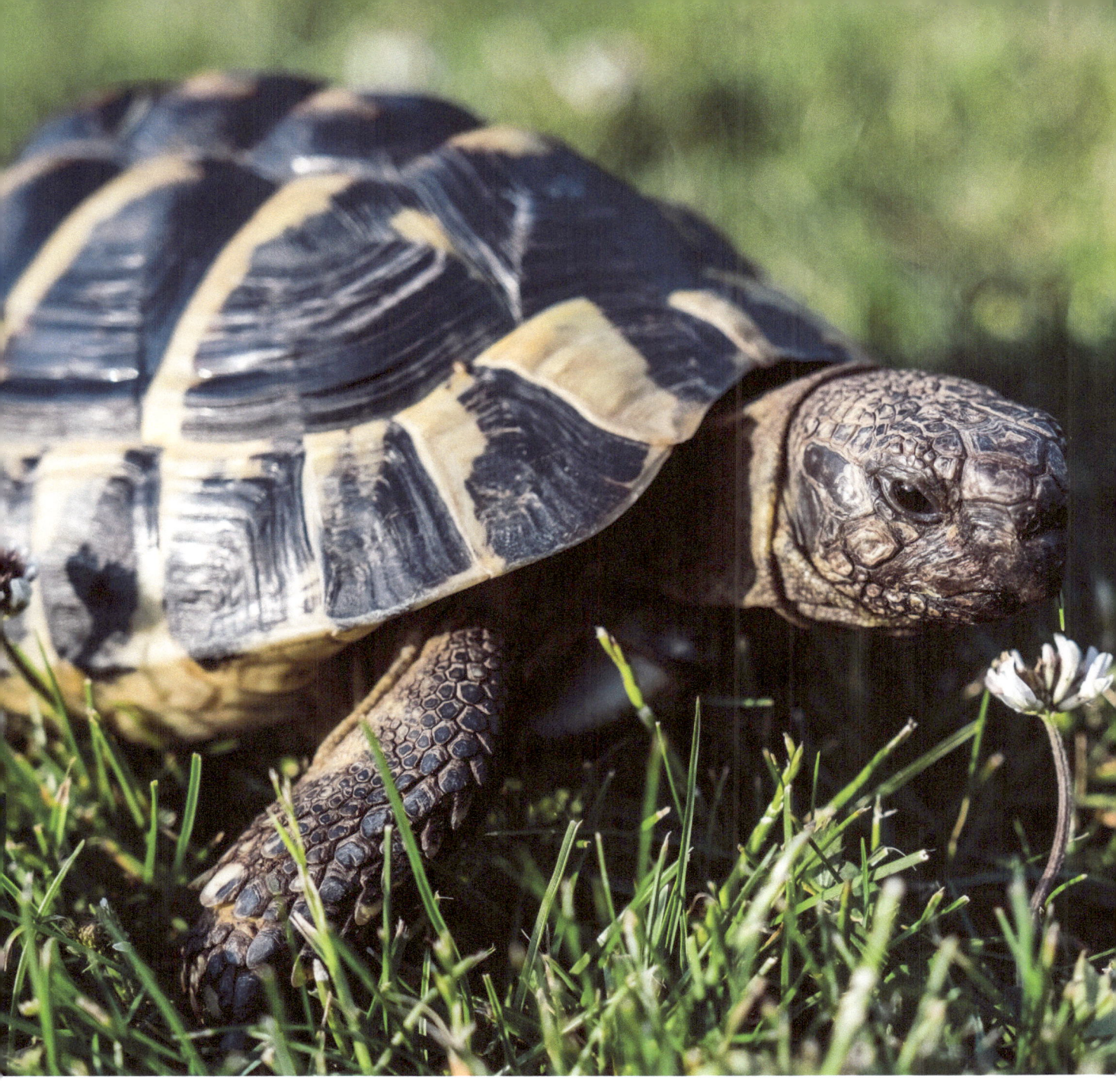

A tortoise

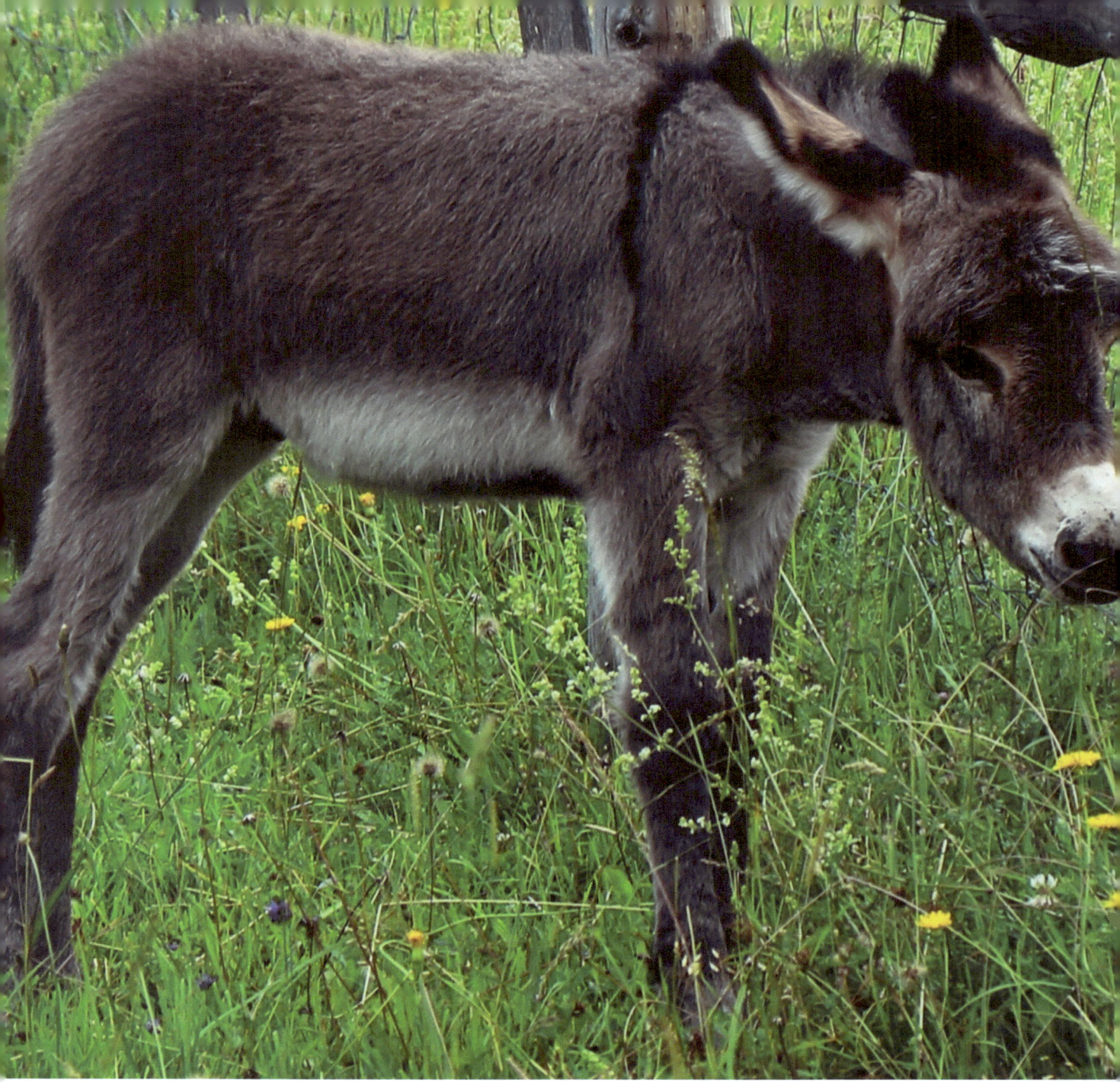

A donkey

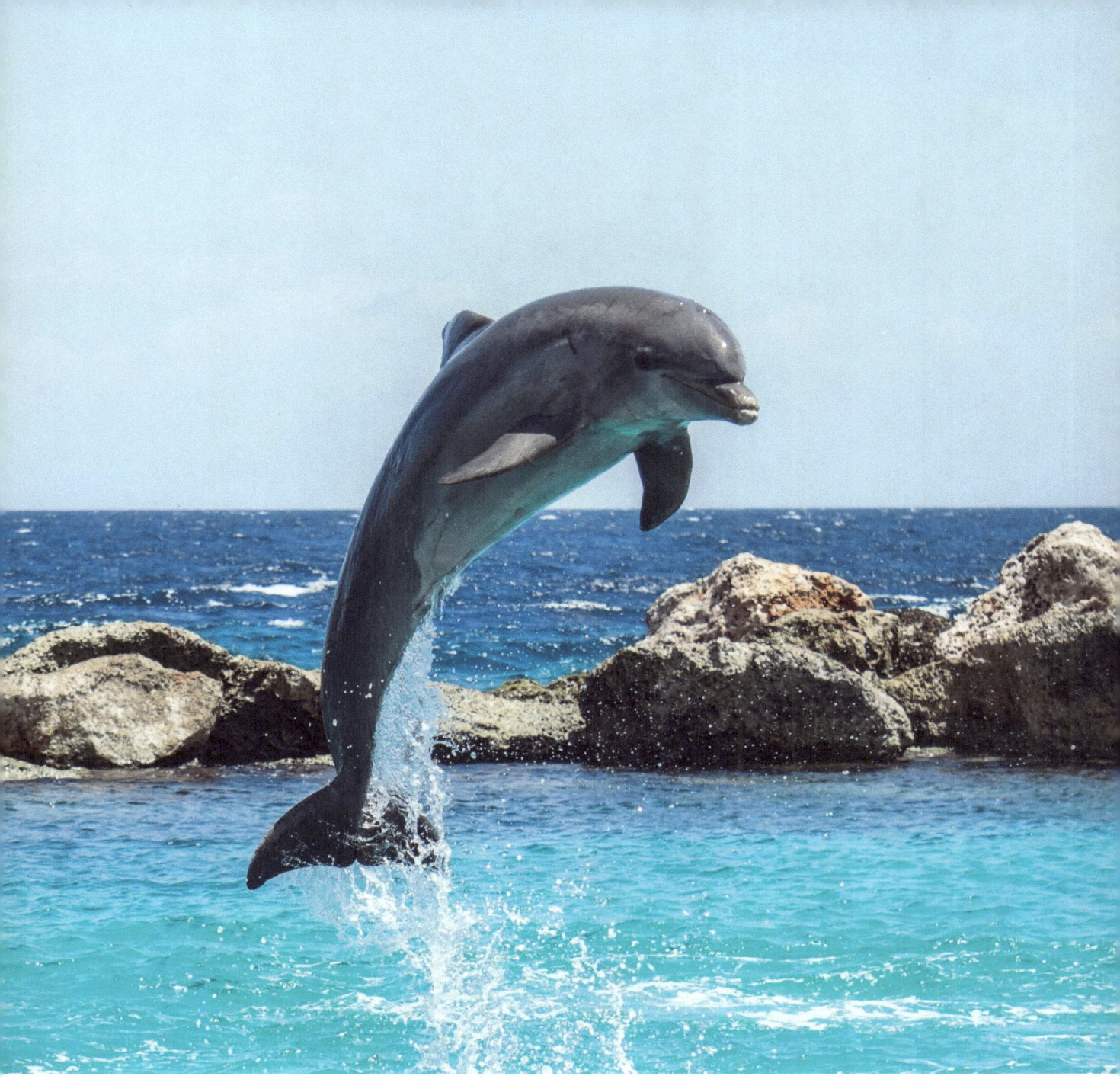

A dolphin

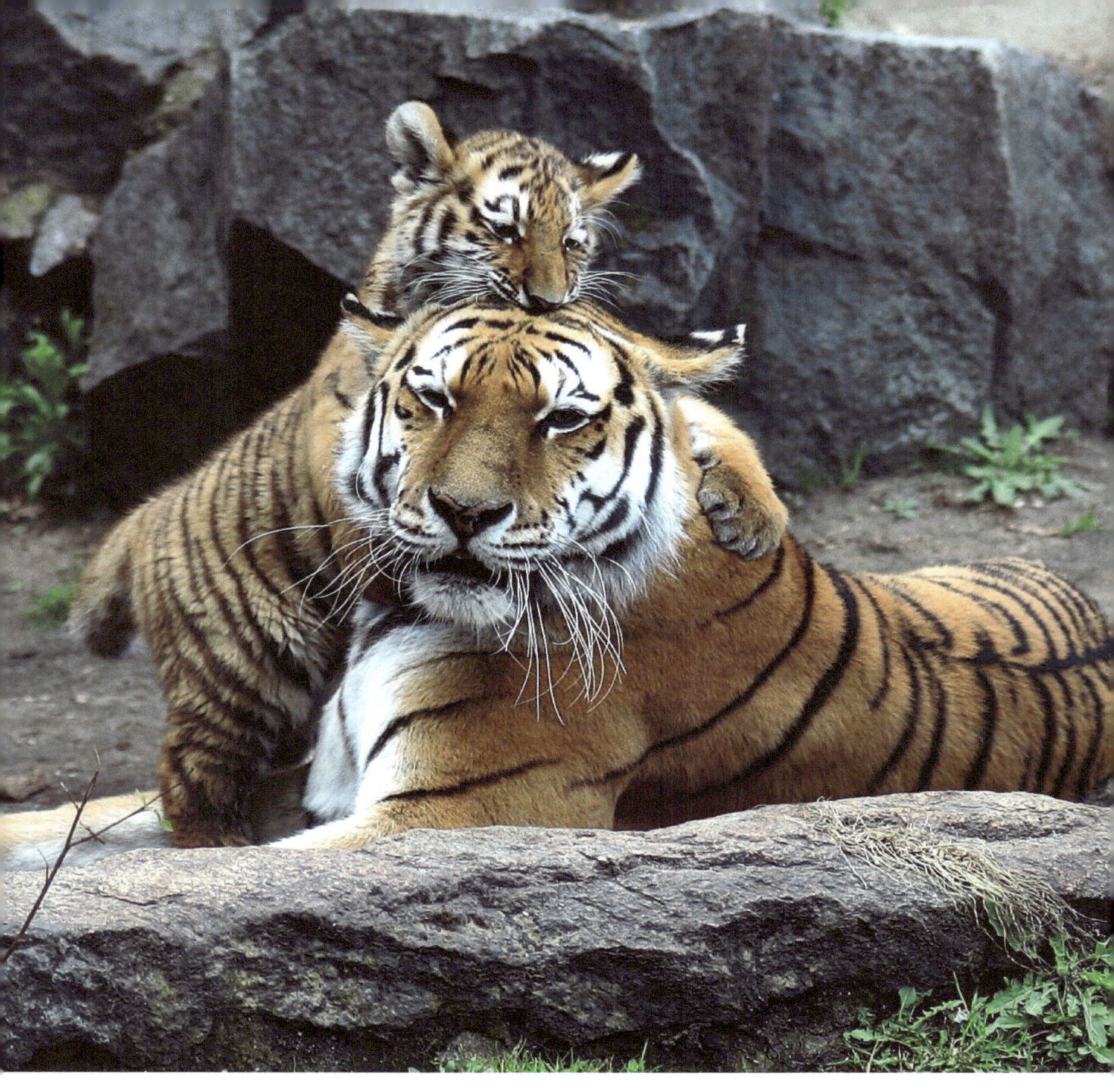

Two tigers

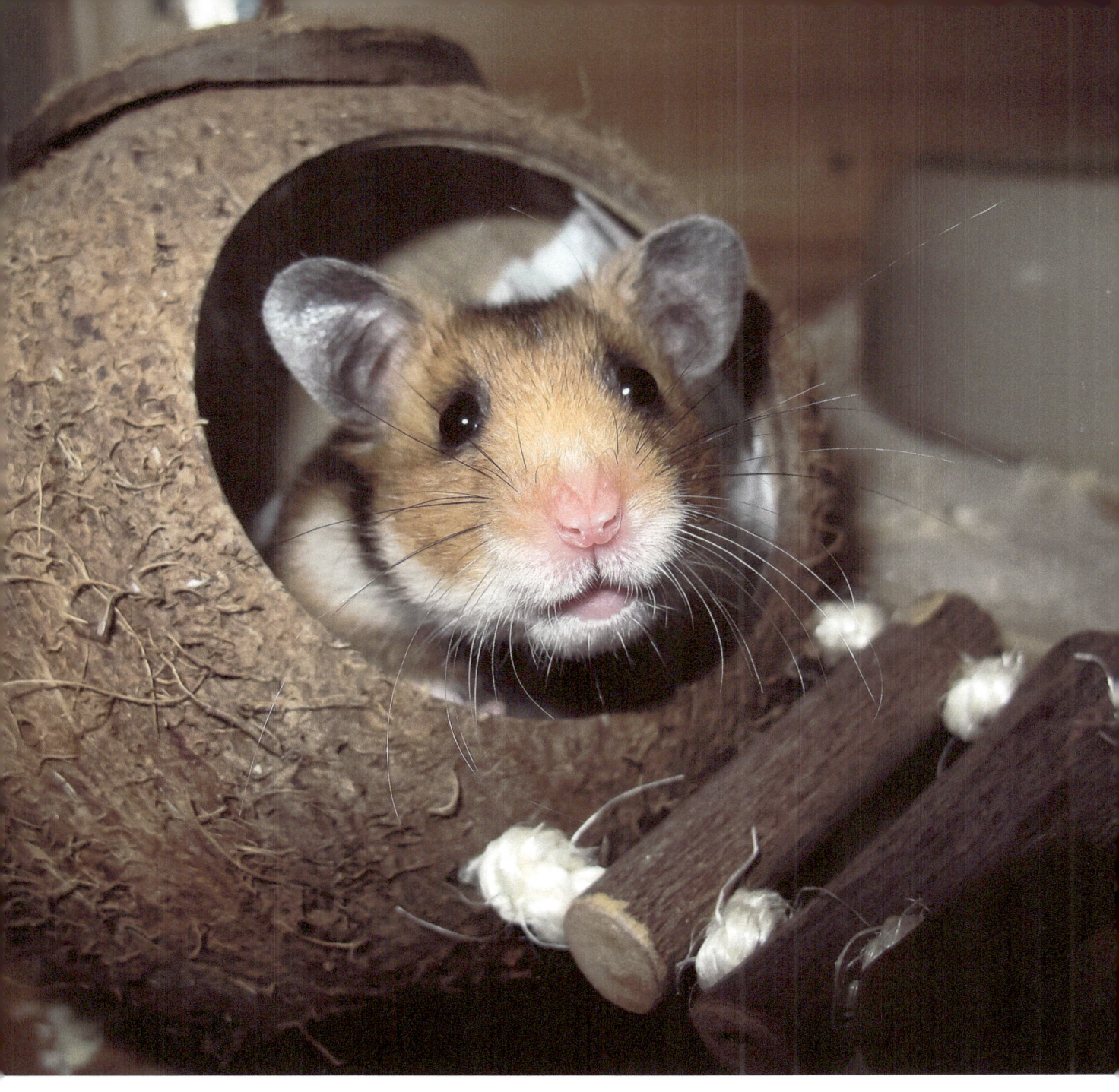

A hamster

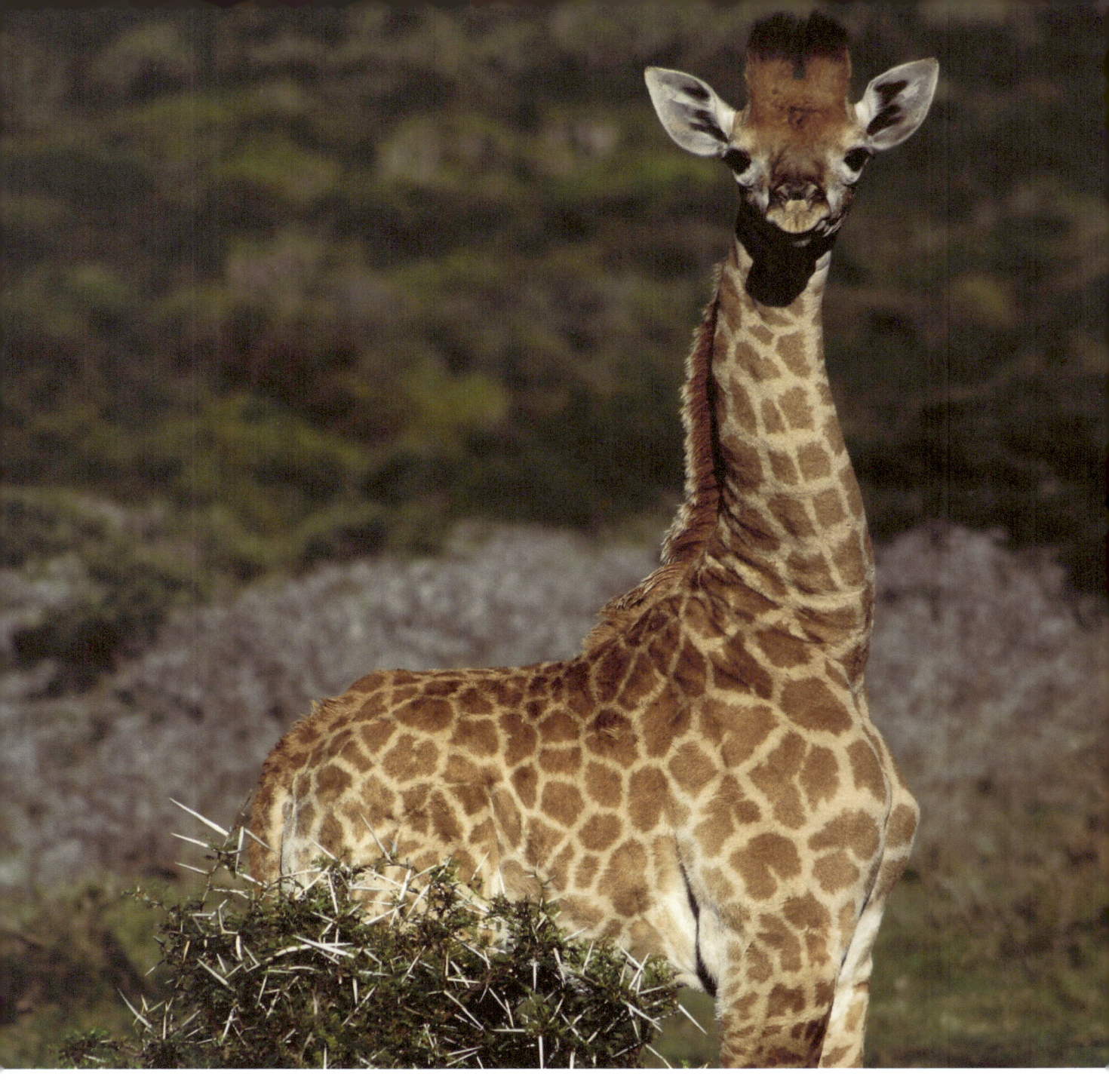

A giraffe

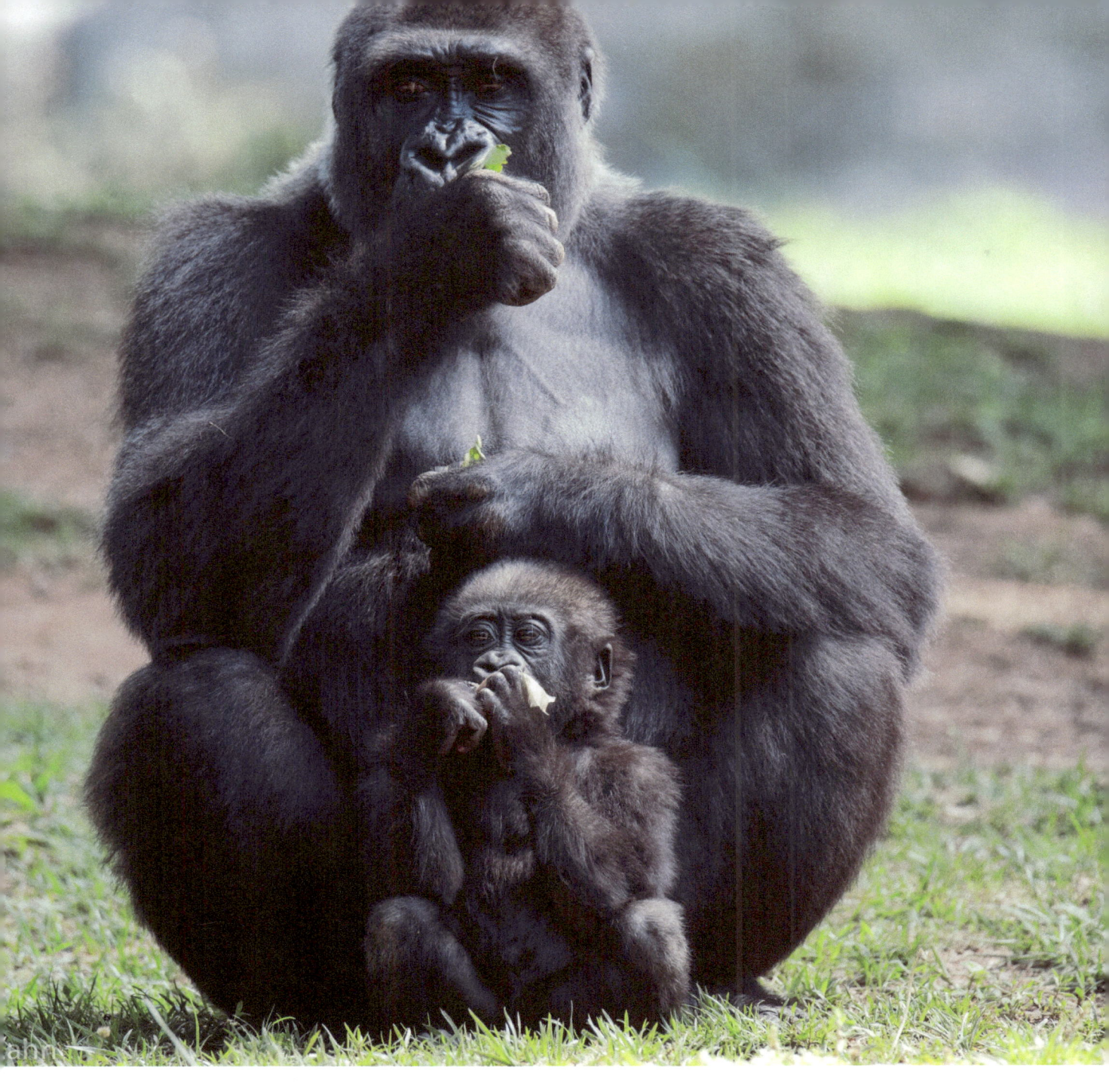

Two gorillas

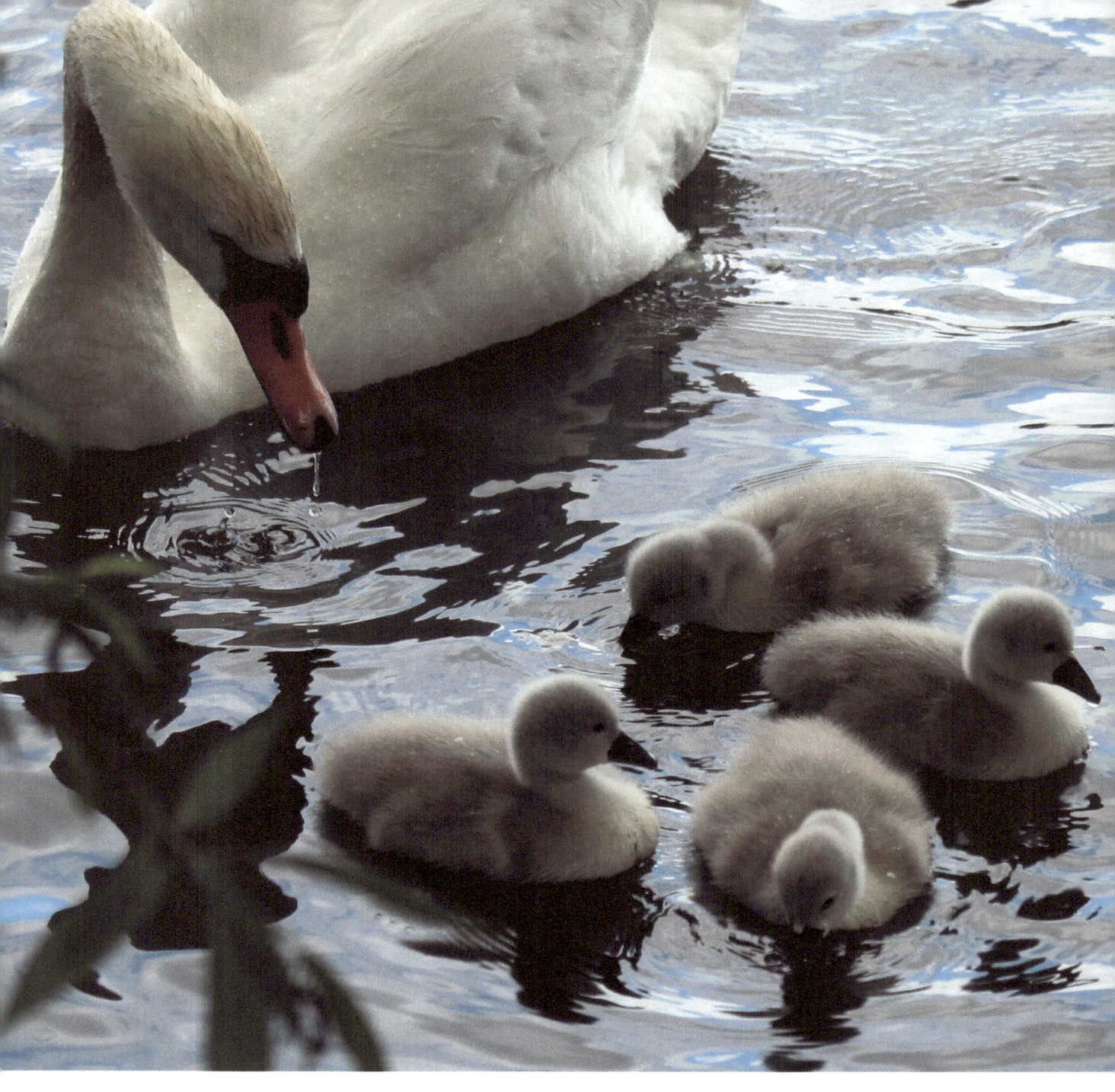

Swans

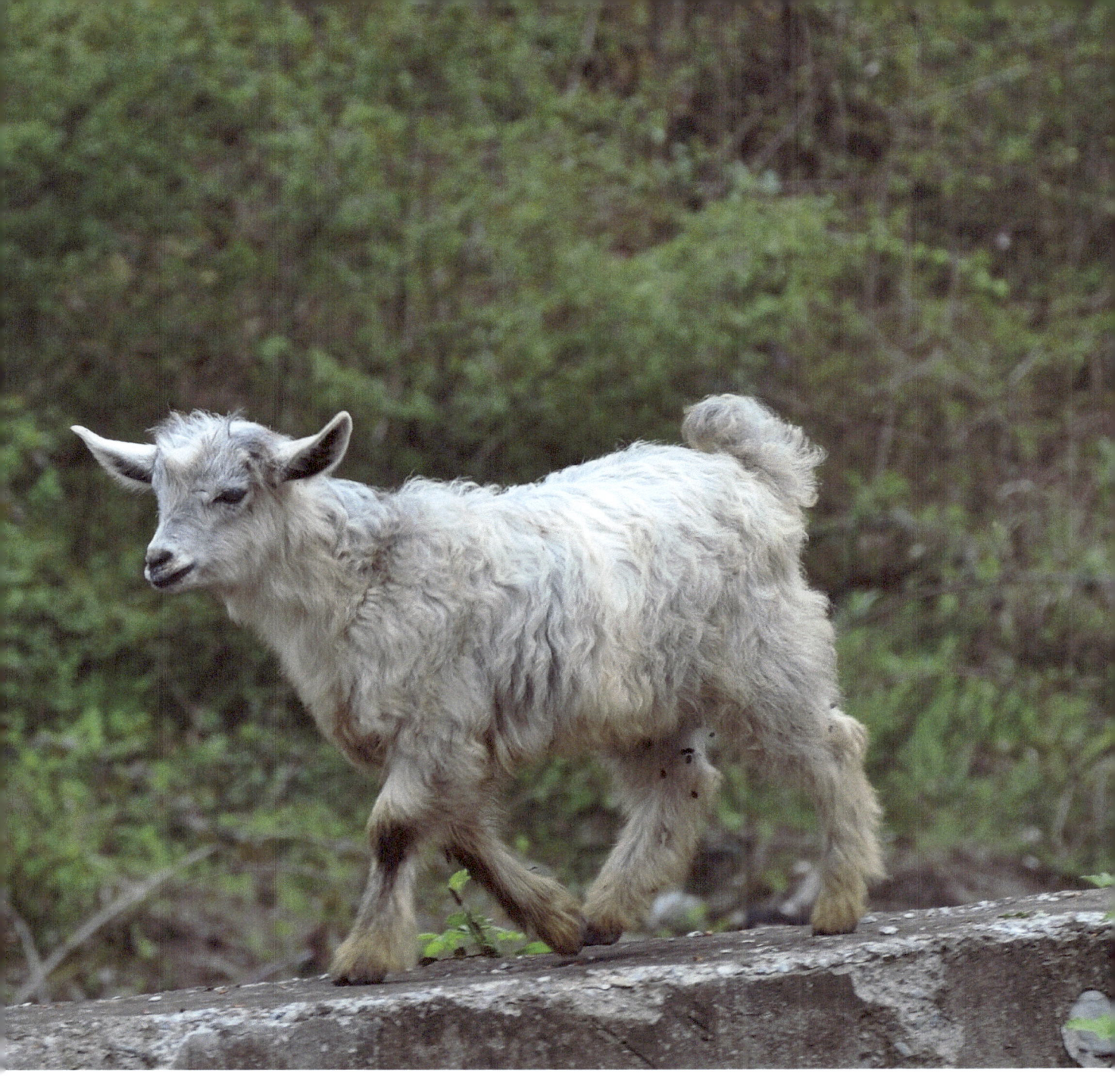

A kid

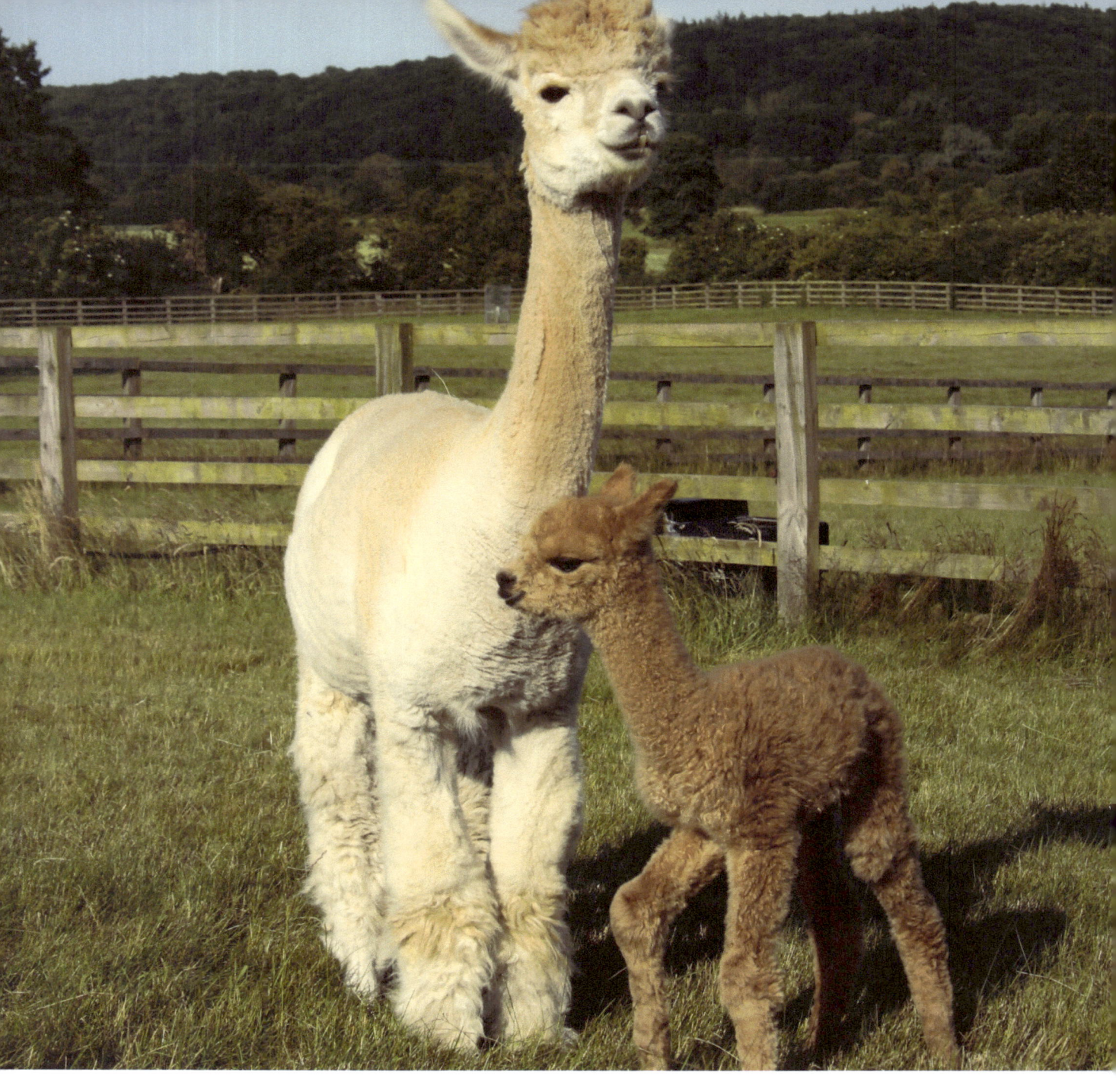

Two llamas

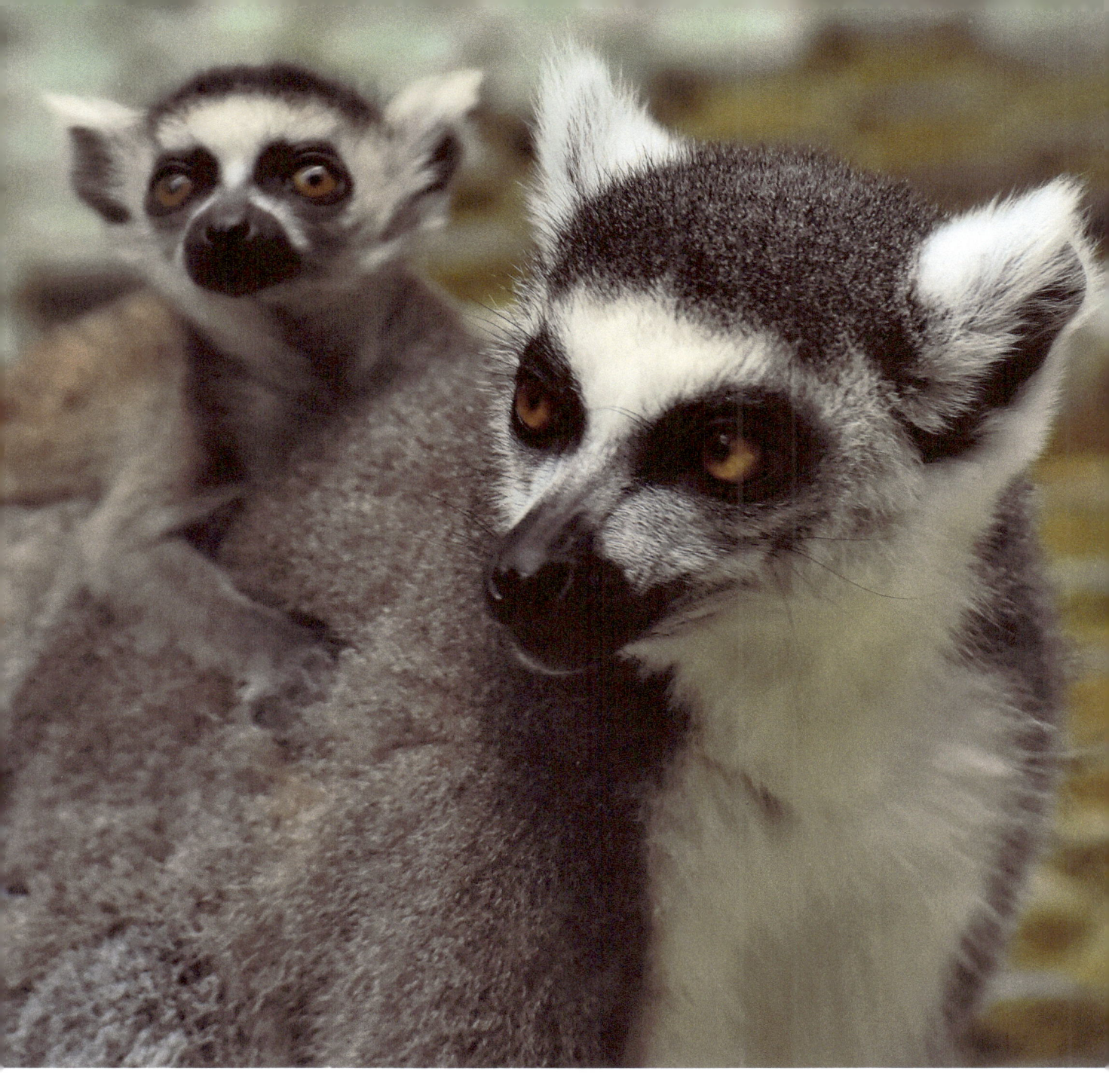

Two lemurs

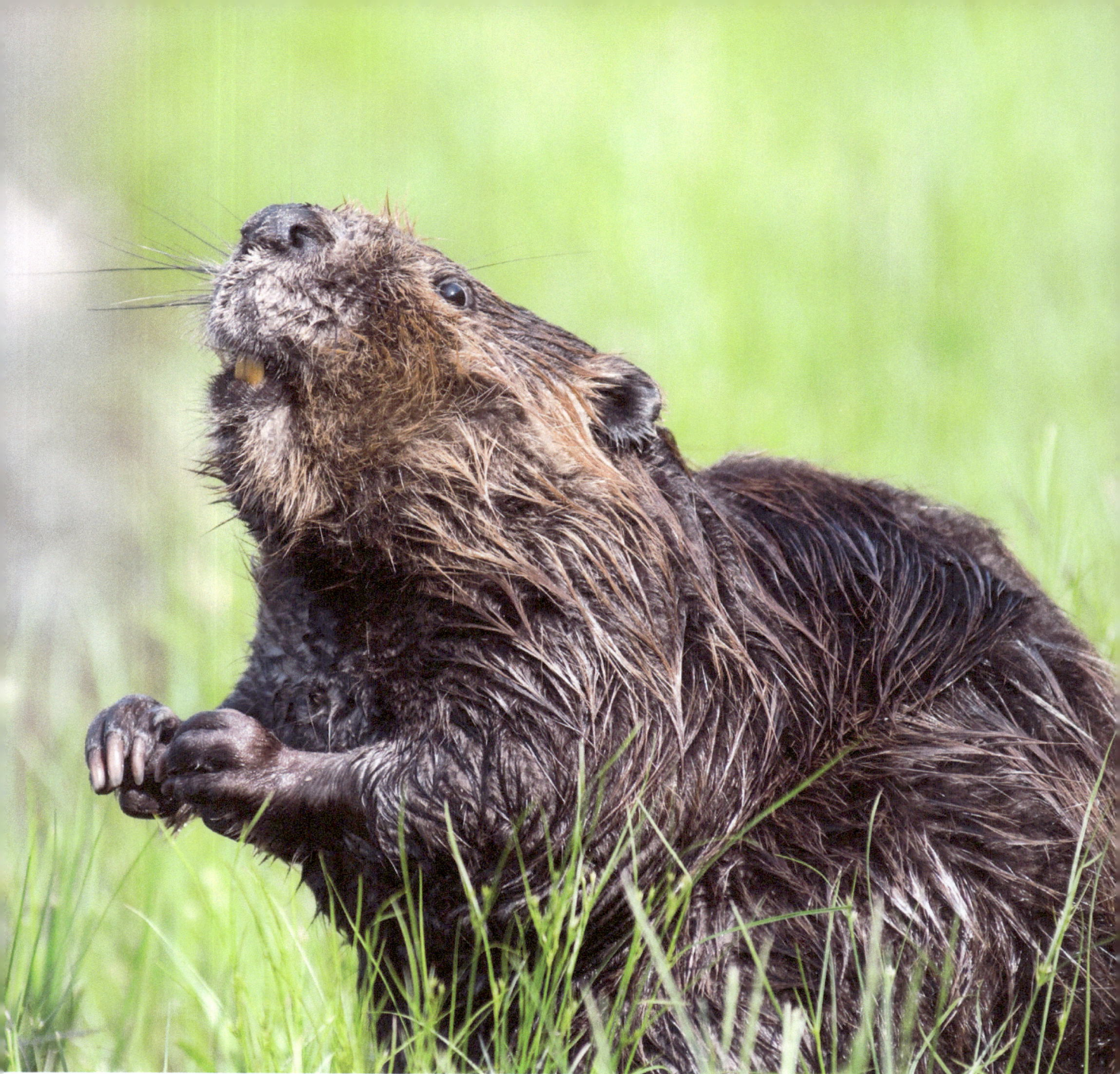

A beaver

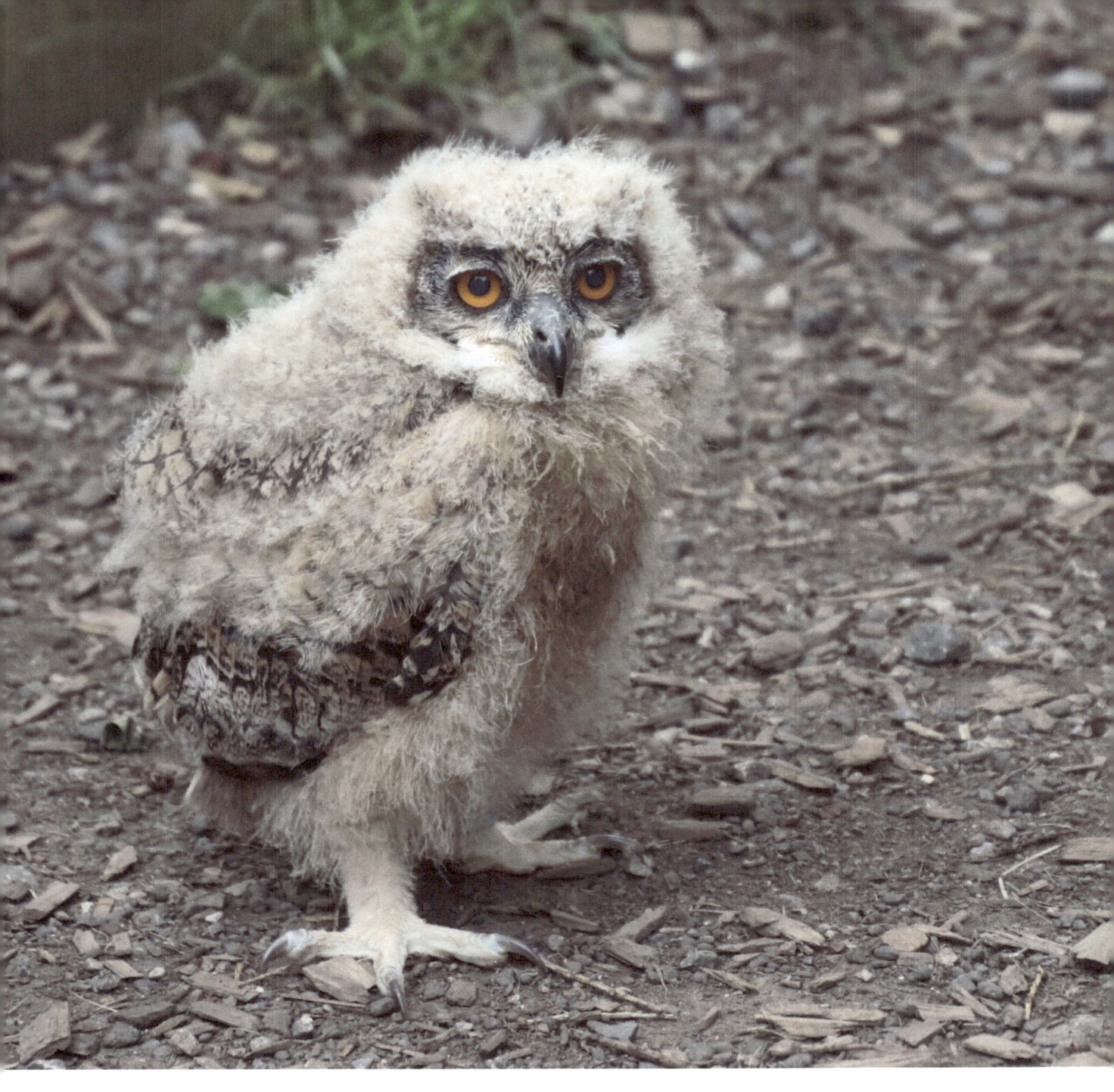

An owl

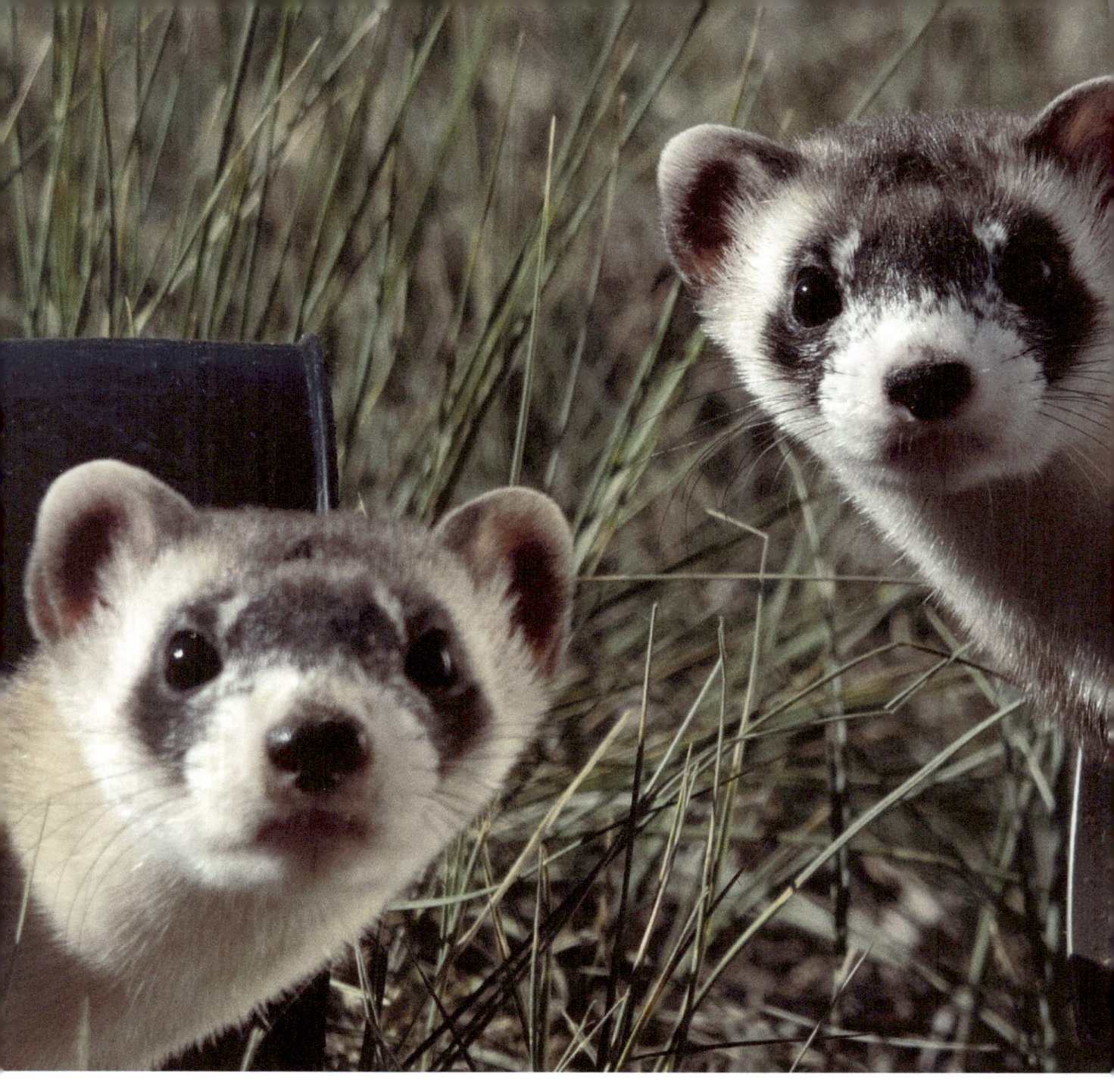

Two ferrets